MW00710922

OTR Exam
Review Manual
Second Edition

Group Natalie
Tuesday 4:30

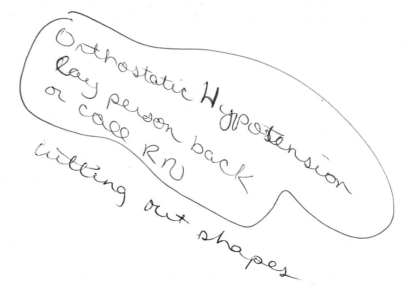

Orthostatic Hypotension
lay person back
or call RN
lifting out shapes

OTR Exam
Review Manual
Second Edition

Karen Sladyk, PhD, OTR/L
Bay Path College
Longmeadow, Massachusetts

with

Signian McGeary, MS, OTR/L
Quinnipiac College
Hamden, Connecticut

Lori G. Sladyk, MS, CSE
Rockville High School
Vernon, Connecticut

Roseanna Tufano, MFT, OTR/L
Quinnipiac College
Hamden, Connecticut

SLACK Incorporated, 6900 Grove Road, Thorofare, NJ 08086-9447

Publisher: John H. Bond
Editorial Director: Amy E. Drummond
Senior Associate Editor: Jennifer J. Cahill
Creative Director: Linda Baker

Copyright © 1998 by SLACK Incorporated

All rights reserved. No part of this book may be reproduced, stored in a retrieval system or transmitted in any form or by any means, electronic, mechanical, photocopying, recording or otherwise, without written permission from the publisher, except for brief quotations embodied in critical articles and reviews.

OTR exam review manual/Karen Sladyk; with Signian McGeary, Lori G. Sladyk, Roseanna Tufano.—2nd ed.
      p. cm.
      Includes bibliographical references.
      ISBN 1-55642-372-1
         1. Occupational therapy—Examinations, questions, etc. 2. Occupational therapy—Outlines, syllabi, etc. I. Sladyk, Karen.
[DNLM: 1. Occupational Therapy—examination questions. WB 18.2 088 1997]
RM735.32.087 1997
615.8'515'076—dc21
DNLM/DLC
for Library of Congress   97-49232

Printed in the United States of America

Published by: SLACK Incorporated
              6900 Grove Road
              Thorofare, NJ 08086-9447 USA
              Telephone: 609-848-1000
              Fax: 609-853-5991
              World Wide Web: http://www.slackinc.com

Contact SLACK Incorporated for more information about other books in this field or about the availability of our books from distributors outside the United States.

Authorization to photocopy items for internal or personal use, or the internal or personal use of specific clients, is granted by SLACK Incorporated, provided that the appropriate fee is paid directly to Copyright Clearance Center, 222 Rosewood Drive, Danvers, MA 01923 USA, 508-750-8400. Prior to photocopying items for educational classroom use, please contact the CCC at the address above. Please reference Account Number 9106324 for SLACK Incorporated's Professional Book Division.
For further information on CCC, check CCC Online at the following address: http://www.copyright.com.

Last digit is print number: 10 9 8 7 6 5 4 3 2 1

Dedication

To every occupational therapy student and the teachers
and clinicians who educate them.

Contents

Contents

Acknowledgments

No book would be complete without thanking all the people behind the scenes. This is true for all of us as well. Lori, Roseanna, Signian, Julie, and I want to thank our families for their support. A special thank you to our friends at SLACK Incorporated, especially Amy Drummond, Debra Christy, and Jennifer Cahill. My friends from the University of Connecticut, Department of Adult and Vocational Education, deserve special thanks for their "of course you can do that" attitude. All the occupational therapy faculty at Quinnipiac College in Hamden, Connecticut, especially Kim Hartmann, Muriel Lerner, Marli Cole, Beth O' Sullivan, and Debra Bowler, deserve recognition for enriching our lives and the classes we teach. Many former OT students, now OTRs, were helpful in the development of this book, including Erika Lund, Wendy Carpenter, Pam Guyette, Rory Marcello, and Jeff Abrahamson. This second edition also contains several review questions written by Christine Negro, OTS. We are especially pleased a student who has not even begun to study for the exam was able to write such dynamic questions. Lastly, a special thank you to all occupational therapy students, past, present, and future, for reminding us what teaching is all about. May this book bring you great success on the exam and may your healing hands touch many hearts and minds.

About the Authors

Karen Sladyk has a BS in Occupational Therapy from Eastern Michigan University, a MS in Community Health from Southern Connecticut State University, and a PhD in Adult and Vocational Education at the University of Connecticut. Karen teaches at Bay Path College in Longmeadow, Massachusetts. Her occupational therapy interests include clinical reasoning and fieldwork. She resides in Vernon, Connecticut in a very old house with two cats. When she is not busy with academic challenges, she enjoys quilt making.

Signian McGeary has 20 years of adult physical disability practice following her degree in Occupational Therapy from Quinnipiac College. Her transition into teaching has resulted in a MS in Adult Education. Her current clinical interests include a research study in hip fractures and outcome studies using the A-one for ADL evaluations. She has studied Mandarin Chinese to prepare for educational clinical exchanges in China with the World Health Organization. Recently, she took eight students to China for a nontraditional Level II fieldwork experience. Her husband, two daughters, and new son-in-law share and support her love of international travel.

Lori G. Sladyk has a BS degree in Social Work from Southern Connecticut State University, a teaching certificate in Special Education, and a MS in Language Arts from Central Connecticut State College. She is currently pursuing an advanced graduate degree in Learning Disabilities at the University of Connecticut. When she is not busy with work and school she is active in community activities with her three sons, Brent, Seth, and Blake. Lori also holds a teaching position (secondary), lives in an old house in Vernon, and enjoys quilt making, but is much different from her sister, Karen, in that she only has one cat.

Roseanna Tufano has a BS degree in Occupational Therapy from Quinnipiac College. She has worked in a variety of psychiatric settings since 1980 as a staff OTR and consultant. She is presently assistant professor at Quinnipiac College where she teaches psychopathology, group dynamics, clinical media, and psychosocial aspects of physical disabilities. Roseanna has recently completed her master's in Marriage and Family Therapy. She resides with her husband, Lou, and their two children, Carissa and Brett. They continue to be her source for love, inspiration, and fun.

Preface

Becoming an OTR is not a simple task. Getting into an occupational therapy program, completing the schooling, the months of fieldwork, and then finally the certification exam takes a lot of time, commitment, and effort. Many of us who are OTRs think occupational therapy is the best career you could choose. This study guide is designed to help you get ready for the last step in becoming an OTR—the certification exam.

This study guide is designed with the student in mind. It is lovingly written by experts in the field of occupational therapy with the sole purpose of helping you get though the studying process and successfully negotiating the certification exam. Although the material is serious, we have attempted to make it light and humorous when possible. To make it easier to read, we have provided the information you need in paragraphs with clear headings.

The book is divided into four main sections: Getting Ready, Study Techniques, Study Questions, and Life After the Exam. The first two chapters deal with a general overview of the examination process. Also included are numerous tools to get yourself organized. The second section includes chapters on content and using your fieldwork experiences to guide your studying. The third section contains 450 study questions set up in the same format as the certification exam. The certification exam is made up of 200 questions with a 4-hour time limit, so our study questions are divided into groups of 50 questions with a time limit of 1 hour. The last section deals with life after the exam and provides some practical advice if things do not go well. We have also included information in the appendices you may find helpful.

In Appendix E, you will find a feedback sheet for us. After you have studied for the exam, we would appreciate a short note from you about this book. Let us know what you liked and did not like about the book. Is there something you wished we had done differently? Future students will benefit from your insights.

Best Wishes,

Karen Sladyk, PhD, OTR/L

SECTION I
Getting Ready

Chapter One

Overview

WHAT TO DO FIRST

Many students preparing for the OTR exam ask the question "What should I do first?" The answer is "It depends." This study guide includes information for every type of person. Where you start depends on how much time you have left to study. In an attempt to give you some structure, let's first look at how much time you have between opening this book for the first time and the next certification exam. The certification exam is given on the third Saturday of March and September. Calculate the time you have until the next exam, and then check the table below for a suggestion of what to do next.

What To Do First	
Time Left Until the Next Exam	*Start Your Reading Here*
6 or more months	Good for you, you have plenty of time to study. Read entire study guide. Study 1 to 2 hours per week.
4 to 5 months	You planned well. Read entire study guide. Begin with 3 to 4 hours per week.
2 to 3 months	No need to panic, you have some time but you must be efficient. Read entire study guide this week. Aim for an hour per day until the study guide is completed. Adjust your study time from there.
About 1 month	Time to get serious. Read entire study guide this week. Aim for at least 1 to 2 hours per day until the study guide is completed. Begin your study plan developed in Chapter Two.
3 weeks	Skip Chapters One and Seven for now. Begin with Chapters Two and Six. Try at least 100 questions in Chapter Five. Adjust your study plan from there.
2 weeks	Complete Chapter Five. Read Chapters Two and Four. Develop a study plan from there.
1 week or less	Complete Chapter Five. Skim Chapters Two and Four for test-taking suggestions.
If you are already an OTR and are using this book for review	If you are taking the exam: Begin with Chapters Five and Six. Skim Chapters Two and Four. If you are not taking the exam but doing a review: Complete Chapters Five and Six.

Assuming you have at least 40 hours of study time ahead of you, the entire study guide is within reach. A good place to start is right here. A little history about the certification process will give you a better understanding of the exam.

CERTIFICATION PROCESS

The National Board for Certification in Occupational Therapy (NBCOT) is a private, nonprofit agency responsible for the development and administration of the certification exam for OTRs. In addition, NBCOT manages the exam for certification of COTAs. Management of each exam requires development of high standards to protect and serve the public. This ensures quality occupational therapy personnel are entering the profession. NBCOT meets the challenge by developing policies and working closely with the development committee with test and measurement experts to ensure quality. Although certification of an OTR may not be required by a few work sites, most governmental, regulatory, insurance, and other agencies use NBCOT examinations as a credential standard. Many state licensing boards require passing the certification exam as the minimum standard for employment.

OTR Examination Question Development

The questions on the OTR certification exam are based on a survey conducted by practicing OTRs and educators to establish the knowledge of entry-level clinicians. The study focused on the skills needed by a new graduate to successfully practice occupational therapy. The study results are used by the Certification Examination Development Committee (CEDC) to develop new exam questions. Expert OTRs from a variety of work settings across the country make up the NBCOT CEDC. The 14 members of this committee are trained in item writing and develop exam questions specific to their content area. All items are rigorously reviewed by CEDC before appearing as examination questions. Item writers use the American Occupational Therapy Association (AOTA) document *Uniform Terminology for Occupational Therapy, Third Edition* (1994) as a basis for terminology. This publication is available in the *American Journal of Occupational Therapy*, November/December 1994, or by calling AOTA at 301-652-2682 (1-800-SAY-AOTA if you are a student member). *Uniform Terminology* is the basis for the content of this study guide.

OTR Examination Administration

The NBCOT contracts with a professional testing company to ensure high standards of reliability and validity in the test development and administration. The professional testing agency is responsible for administering and scoring the exam as well as reporting the results to the student. Each OTR certification exam is a unique combination of exam items pulled from a data bank of possible questions. The data banks for COTAs and OTRs are kept separate and the questions are never used in both exams. NBCOT provides a list of content area and the percentage of weight for each area to the test taker ahead of the exam. This outline ensures consistency between the tests over time.

Application for the OTR Examination

The program director at your school will send your name and address to NBCOT when you become eligible to sit for the examination. Your program director will give you a postcard to mail in for exam information. NBCOT will send you a candidate's handbook that will outline the certification process. Inside the handbook will be an application. Follow the rules of the application carefully, including the policies for fees.

OTR Examination Structure

Each exam has 200 multiple choice questions. Each question will have four possible choices labeled A through D. There are no "all of the above" or combination choices on the OTR exam.

The penalty for leaving an answer blank is the same as an incorrect answer, so be sure to fill in your best guess for all items. Choose only one answer for each question and fill in your answer by coloring the appropriate circle with a number two pencil. The examination will be scored by the testing agency and then reviewed by CEDC to look for flawed questions.

After flawed questions are removed, criterion-referenced scoring will be used to calculate the passing score. This means that those people above the criterion score will pass the certification examination and those below will not.

Your score is not compared to other people who took the exam, but simply compared to the minimum passing level to be an entry-level occupational therapist. Test takers who need special accommodations due to a disability (e.g., visual, hearing, health, or orthopedic impairment or learning, emotional, or multiple disabilities) will be provided with services as outlined in the Americans with Disabilities Act. Information on special accommodations is located in the candidate's handbook from NBCOT. It is important that you provide the documentation necessary and follow the specific process in the handbook.

STUDYING IDEAS

Now that you understand NBCOT and the certification process, it is time to begin to make your study plan. Chapter Two of this book covers your personal study plan in great detail, however, let us briefly look at some ideas you may find helpful.

Study groups: Studying a large amount of material with a group of people can be easier and more efficient. However, not all study groups are effective. You may have experienced a group project in school where one or more participants did not do their fair share. This often leads to resentment and hurt feelings. If you plan to form a study group, ask people you are *certain* will actively participate. If you are asked to join a study group, be sure you have a clear understanding of the group's goals and expectations. In any case, be sure to allow some time at the beginning of the first session to allow everyone an opportunity to share goals and expectations. If someone feels he or she cannot participate, allow the student to decline with dignity.

Exam review conferences: Many occupational therapy schools offer a 1- or 2-day conference to review for the exam. You can call AOTA or an area occupational therapy school to see if one is available.

Lecture notes: Even though you may have had one class that you did not like, the faculty at your school have provided you with a global education in occupational therapy. AOTA requires all occupational therapy programs to meet minimum essentials to receive or maintain the school's accreditation. Your occupational therapy program has met the essential components. This means that your classes provided you with at least the minimum information needed to pass the exam and become a practicing OTR. That said, you should have everything you need to know about occupational therapy written down in your class lecture notes. Reviewing your notes is one of the most effective ways to study for the certification exam.

Textbooks: It would be impossible (and we do not recommend) for you to reread your textbooks from cover to cover. Even if you did not sell them back to the bookstore, reading your textbooks in their entirety is not an effective use of study time.

It **is** appropriate to read your textbooks in the areas that you are weak in. We recommend that you read only the textbook sections in which you need a detailed review. Use your notes from class to provide a basic study outline and refer to the textbooks for more detail. Be sure to save your textbooks for your professional needs after the exam.

We would also like to call your attention to the appendices of this book. We have provided information that you may find helpful as you study for the exam. In Appendix A, you will find a list of suggested occupational therapy references. Do not worry if you have never had a particular textbook in your classes. The suggestions are comprehensive to provide broad coverage of the material on the exam; however, your faculty have chosen an excellent blend of textbooks for you. In addition to the reference list, we have provided a list of abbreviations in Appendix B that you may find helpful. Appendix C contains suggested books to further develop study and test-taking techniques. All of this information is designed to help you get ready for the "big day."

EXAM DAY

The day of the exam will be filled with much nervous energy. It is best to plan ahead to enhance the chances of a smooth day. The old advice of a good night's sleep and eating well before any test is especially true for taking the exam. You may want to try a dry run to the test site prior to exam day if you are unfamiliar with the location. If you are traveling on an exam day that might have bad weather, listen to the weather report and allow extra time to get to the exam site if needed. If you are driving, fill your gas tank the day before the exam.

Wear comfortable clothes but keep in mind the season and weather. Layered clothing will allow you to adjust your clothing if the room is too warm or cool. If your hair is long, tie it back but avoid wearing a baseball cap or any other type of hat that blocks your eyes from the exam proctors.

Have a bag ready to take with you as you leave for the test site. Include the following items in your bag:

1. A map to the test site if you are unfamiliar with the location
2. Change for a pay phone to call for directions or help if needed
3. A watch
4. A minimum of three sharpened number two pencils
5. A clean eraser
6. Photo identification
7. Tissues
8. A snack high in carbohydrates (i.e., a bagel) for long-term thinking power (eat before entering the testing room as food is not allowed during the exam)
9. Chewing gum, if needed
10. Reading glasses, if you use them
11. Your admission ticket

Once you arrive at the test site, get in line to register. While waiting to enter the exam room you may want to use the restroom. If you are anxious, avoid talking to people who will make you feel more nervous. Find a quiet space to relax. Do not study or review notes. This is the time to focus on relaxing. Talk with friends and arrange to meet for lunch or dinner after the exam to catch up on news.

COUNTDOWN CALENDAR

A blank calendar is provided to help you organize your last month before the exam. Use this calendar to chart your goals and study plans. Begin by entering the month (March or September) and year you will take the exam. Enter the dates in each box. The exam is always given on the

Countdown Calendar						
Sunday	*Monday*	*Tuesday*	*Wednesday*	*Thursday*	*Friday*	*Saturday*
						Map and Check Route to Exam
						EXAM DAY

third Saturday. Enter the exam date and fill in the other dates on the calendar. Remove the calendar from the book and post it in a prominent place. Once you have a dated calendar of your goals, can begin to develop your study plans in Chapter Two.

SUMMARY

Beginning to study for the certification exam can be overwhelming. Information on where to start is provided in this chapter. The role of NBCOT, and the history and process of the exam are reviewed to help you understand the exam. General study techniques and a countdown calendar are provided to guide you through your exam preparation. Information for a smooth exam day is also included.

SECTION II
Study Techniques

Chapter Two

How to Study for the Exam

GETTING STARTED

Congratulations! Obviously you care enough about your upcoming exam to purchase and read this book. Okay, so you couldn't part with the money, but you asked your parents to buy it for you. Even if you *borrowed* this book, your intentions are still good. You've done well enough in college to get to this point. You don't need a "how to" study guide because you have already been successful. However, you may wish to look at your current study habits and determine whether you can be a more efficient learner. Perhaps there is a study technique that you have not thought of, or a memory strategy that can benefit you. The purpose of this chapter is to help you select the study techniques that will benefit you.

You are in charge. No one will know if you are in your room studying or reading a magazine. You are responsible for your study plan. Studying may be a burden, but it is a light one to bear considering the alternatives: having fun, going out, watching TV, etc. Oh all right! There are other things you could be doing, but you may not get the same result. Effective studying will give you satisfaction, peace of mind, and added confidence. You will know that no matter what the outcome is, you have done your best and can hold your head high.

Remember, you are a unique individual. Do not waste time comparing yourself to others studying for the exam. Your experiences and personal situations are different than others'. Accept your personal strengths and weaknesses, and develop a plan of attack based on your needs. Listen to others' good suggestions but stick to the plan that will benefit you. Be honest in your own assessments, and be willing to admit if something is not working. Evaluate your plan regularly to see if you are obtaining the results you intended. If not, modify your plan based on what you need.

Take the time now to make a plan. Even if it is a lousy one, you are heading in the right direction. You can always change it later, but at least relieve some stress by making some decisions. The following pages will assist you in assessing your current learning preferences in order to develop an effective plan.

FINDING YOUR BEST LEARNING STYLE

Learning styles refer to the way people take in, store, and retrieve information. Some people learn and remember best by hearing, while others learn by writing. You may have a preference for one style or modality or you may find that a combination of styles works best for you. Take the following inventory to help determine your strongest learning preference. Check the following characteristics that apply to you.

LEARNING STYLE CHARACTERISTICS CHECKLIST

1. ___ When I have a problem, I usually tell someone right away.
2. ___ I keep a journal.
3. ___ I often take notes, although I do not always refer to them.
4. ___ I take good notes and then rewrite them at a later time.

5. ☒ I read in my free time.
6. ✓ I have the TV on even if I am not watching it.
7. ___ I have good intentions of writing to people but usually call instead.
8. ___ I often shut my eyes to help me concentrate.
9. ___ When studying or solving a problem, I pace back and forth.
10. ___ I would rather hear a book on audiocassette than read it myself.
11. ___ Forget the cassette, I would rather wait until it comes out on film.
12. ✓ I prefer reading the newspaper to watching the news on TV.
13. ✓ I prefer to study in a quiet setting.
14. ✓ To remember a spelling, I "see" the word in my mind.
15. ___ I would prefer an oral exam to a written one.
16. ✓ I prefer a multiple choice format on a test.
17. ___ I would rather do a project than write a paper.
18. ✓ I would rather give an oral report than a written one.
19. ___ I remember better what I read rather than what I hear.
20. ✓ I keep a personal organizer.
21. ___ I reread my notes several times.
22. ___ I would rather take notes from the text than attend a lecture on the material.
23. ✓ I often "talk to myself."
24. ___ I learn best when I study with a partner.
25. ✓ I can locate a passage that I have read by "seeing it."
26. ✓ I find it hard to sit still when I study.
27. ___ If I forgot why I walked in the kitchen, I retrace my steps from the bedroom.
28. ___ Once in bed for the night, I shut my eyes and plan the next day.
29. ___ I cannot clean unless the music is on.
30. ✓ I would rather read directions than have someone tell me about them.
31. ___ I can put something together as long as the directions are written.

SCORING THE CHECKLIST

Compare your answers from your checklist to the checklist below. Circle the letters that correspond to your answers.

1. **S** When I have a problem, I usually tell someone right away.
2. **W** I keep a journal.
3. **MW** I often take notes, although I do not always refer to them.
4. **W** I take good notes and then rewrite them at a later time.
5. **R** I read in my free time.
6. **L** I have the TV on even if I am not watching it.
7. **S** I have good intentions of writing to people but usually call instead.
8. **V** I often shut my eyes to help me concentrate.
9. **M** When studying or solving a problem, I pace back and forth.
10. **L** I would rather hear a book on audiocassette than read it myself.
11. **V** Forget the cassette, I would rather wait until it comes out on film.
12. **R** I prefer reading the newspaper to watching the news on TV.
13. **L** I prefer to study in a quiet setting.
14. **V** To remember a spelling, I "see" the word in my mind.
15. **S** I would prefer an oral exam to a written one.

16. **V**   I prefer a multiple choice format on a test.
17. **M**   I would rather do a project than write a paper.
18. **S**   I would rather give an oral report than a written one.
19. **R**   I remember better what I read rather than what I hear.
20. **W**   I keep a personal organizer.
21. **R**   I reread my notes several times.
22. **W**   I would rather take notes from the text than attend a lecture on the material.
23. **SL**   I often "talk to myself."
24. **SL**   I learn best when I study with a partner.
25. **V**   I can locate a passage that I have read by "seeing it."
26. **M**   I find it hard to sit still when I study.
27. **M**   If I forgot why I walked in the kitchen, I retrace my steps from the bedroom.
28. **V**   Once in bed for the night, I shut my eyes and plan the next day.
29. **L**   I cannot clean unless the music is on.
30. **R**   I would rather read directions than have someone tell me about them.
31. **R**   I can put something together as long as the directions are written.

Tally the number of S, W, M, R, L, and V responses and record the total in the following table.

S	W	M	R	L	V
3	2	2	8	3	3

If you have three or more responses of one letter, you most likely have a strong preference for that learning style. Most people have at least one strength, but you may have more than one.

RESULTS

Speaking (S): Three or more checks in this area indicates a preference for learning information by saying it. You may wish to read your notes and text aloud, or at least the chapter headings. It may be beneficial for you to have a study partner, or to speak into a tape recorder and play your tape back. You may ask someone to listen to you as you explain a principle. After reviewing information, play the part of a teacher by asking questions aloud. Repeat concepts aloud and ask questions of others.

Writing (W): Take notes from readings. Rewrite your notes on paper or index cards. Make tests for yourself and take them. Write notes in the margins of your text and notebooks.

Manipulative (M): Often thought of as the kinesthetic modality, learning occurs best by "doing." If you have this type of preference, make a model, map, or diagram of the information you need to learn. Write information on a black/white board. Carry index cards with the information you are trying to learn with you and pull out the cards while you are walking, exercising, or cooking dinner. Draw answers in the air as you try to memorize information. Move your lips while reading or thinking.

Reading (R): Read and reread information if this is your preferred learning style. Ask to borrow other students' notes so you can read them and fill in any information you may have missed. Highlight text passages to easily locate information. Read chapter titles, headings, and summaries.

Listening (L): You would benefit from having a study group or at least a partner. To the extent possible, have others read to you. Tape lectures and review sessions whenever possible. Make review tapes for yourself and listen to them. Read and repeat information aloud after you have read or heard it. Call classmates and have them read their notes to you or quiz you over the phone.

Visualizing (V): If this is your learning strength, you learn best by picturing information in your head. You are apt to "see" a page of information. It is to your benefit to study, shut your eyes, and then recall the information. Take note of the way the information is written, as well as the shape, color, and size of the paper. This will help you recall the information later. Also picture yourself taking the exam, walking in, and calmly sitting down. This will help steady your nerves.

Often it is beneficial for you to study in more than one way. Remember, your learning profile is unique and just because your friend studies best when listening to music does not mean that the same will apply to you. Take a moment to inventory your strengths and develop a plan based on the way you learn best.

GETTING ORGANIZED TO STUDY

How much time do you have to study, or how much time are you willing to give based on your work schedule, information remembered from classes, anxiety level, and other commitments? Fill out the following time log to visually see how you have been spending your time. If possible, do this for several days, including Saturday and Sunday.

Time Log			
Day:			
6:00-7:00 a.m.			
7:00-8:00			
8:00-9:00			
9:00-10:00			
10:00-11:00			
11:00-12:00 noon			
12:00-1:00 p.m.			
1:00-2:00			
2:00-3:00			
3:00-4:00			
4:00-5:00			
5:00-6:00			
6:00-7:00			
7:00-8:00			
8:00-9:00			
9:00-10:00			
10:00-11:00			

Based on how your time is usually spent, what available time do you have for studying? Will you be better off studying for a block of time in the afternoon, or for several chunks throughout the day? Perhaps your schedule is such that you can only study on weekends. How much time can you commit to studying during your free time? Based on the amount of time you have, make a plan of when you are going to study. (You can always modify it later.)

Study Time Commitments

Next, make a list of the supplies you will need for studying. This may sound nerdy, but it is a lot more fun studying if you have colored index cards and a candy supply.

Study Supplies	
Suggested Study Supplies	*Your List of Study Supplies*
Reference books (DSM-IV, texts, guides, dictionary, etc.)	
Assorted colored index cards	
Index cards on a wire	
Notetabs	
Assorted colored highlighters	
Timer/clock	
Goal sheet: long- and short-term	
Writing instruments	
Tissues	
Water or beverage	
Tape recorder	
Lined/unlined paper	
Snacks or treats	
Tools of the trade (goniometer, etc.)	
Class notes, prior exams if available	
Rabbit's foot or other good luck charms	

Stock your study area with the supplies you determined were needed. If you travel to the library, or study in several different places, prepare a bag with your supplies so you will always have them at hand. Note: if you have run out of snacks more than three times, you need to re-evaluate your priorities!

Now that you have determined when you will study and what you need to begin, you are ready to make a plan of attack. Begin by developing a goal sheet for yourself. Examine the sample on the next page as a guideline for your goal sheet.

Sample Goal Sheet			
Outcome Goal: *To pass NBCOT exam and become an OTR*			
Current Date	*Objectives*	*Target Completion Date*	*Revision of Goals or Progress Notes*
11/30	Complete 30 questions from review manual	11/30	Done. Got 23 correct.
12/1	Photocopy Amy's notes on TBI; give her copy of my SCI notes	12/2	
12/4	Read chapter summaries in textbooks	12/4	Took longer than expected. Finished 12/5.
12/6	Make flashcards/ vocab cards	12/6	Ran out of cards. Go shopping by 12/8.
12/9	Tape record content outline from text	12/11	Done. Victorious!
12/10	Finish vocab cards	12/10	Done. Pat self on back.
12/12	Highlight vocab in text	12/15	Finished 12/13. See a movie.
12/15	Reorganize notebook	12/16	No interest. Try again.
12/16	Form a study group	12/18	No problem.
12/17	Reorganize notebook	12/18	Watched TV instead.
12/19	Reorganize notebook	12/19	Maybe tomorrow.

Now complete your goal sheet.

Goal Sheet			
Outcome Goal:			
Current Date	*Objectives*	*Target Completion Date*	*Revision of Goals or Progress Notes*
1/11/00	Complete 30 quest	1/11/00	

Review and revise your plan of attack often. If nothing else, remove the sheet from the book and post it where it will remind you that you do have a goal in mind. Be flexible. Your great aunt may stop over (and you know what that means) or you may find yourself completing goals ahead of schedule.

Make goals reasonable. It is unrealistic to expect yourself to complete 300 review questions in an hour, yet completing five vocabulary flashcards per week is no great accomplishment. Base your goals on the amount of overall time you have (and are willing) to study. Chapter One has a countdown calendar to help set your goals.

SPECIFIC STUDY AND TEST SKILLS

Reading comprehension: Points on the exam are not awarded for how long you study, your effort, or the amount of pages you read. Generally grades are earned by knowing the correct information. It is quite important then that you have good comprehension of the material you are reading. Below are suggestions to aid in understanding your reading material.
1. Preview the chapter you are about to read by scanning the title, headings, introduction, summary, and, on occasion, the topic sentence in each paragraph. This can also be helpful to review a chapter or passage you have already read.
2. Take regular breaks to review mentally what you have read.
3. Turn topic sentences into questions.
4. Answer these in your head or jot them down for later review.
5. Read the material carefully, checking your understanding as you go along.

Note taking: Taking notes on material that you are studying can be beneficial. Remember, even if you never review the notes you take, the process of jotting them down can be helpful. Outlining with highlighters may help zero in on the main idea. If this method works well for you, use a different colored marker to highlight the details or supporting ideas. Reread your highlighted passages. Class notes can be highlighted as well as textbooks. Use margin notes to organize what you have read. Pay attention to key words or write questions in the margin for later review. Margin notes will help avoid wasted time searching for an answer because the explanation will be right there.

Another way to take notes on important material is to jot down information in a separate notebook. Again, this is particularly helpful for those who learn best kinesthetically. Note taking should always be done by using phrases rather than complete sentences. Make an informal outline by writing down the main idea from a passage and several supporting details under the idea. Always jot down the page number or source of information so you can refer back to it if needed.

If you have found that you remember information best by picturing the words on a page or by writing, then you might consider mapping as a note taking strategy. Draw a circle in the middle of your page and write the main idea in it. Write the major points regarding your main topic on connecting lines. This might include information such as causes and effects, or symptoms and treatments. Add lines to your major points to connect minor details. See Figure 2-1 for an occupational therapy mapping example.

Lastly, notes can be written on index cards. Put one key concept on each notecard with supporting details. Reference your card so you know where to find additional information should you have a question. Write down pertinent vocabulary to the concept on your card. If there is a definition associated with your concept, write that on the back of your card so you can test yourself. One advantage to using notecards is the opportunity to put a few in your pocket to review when you are waiting for your ride, or to stick on your mirror while you blow dry your hair, or to view on the refrigerator as you contemplate a snack.

Memory strategies: Comprehending the material you hear and read is one thing, but memorizing it is another. Fortunately, most of what is asked of us deals more with integrating and applying information rather than memorizing long lists of terms. However, there are occasions when you will be responsible for producing an exact definition, listing the components of a subject, or remembering several general concepts. If you can recite the alphabet, then you should be able to remember just about anything. Consider all the similar sounding letters in the alphabet (B, C, D, E, G, P, T, V, Z), yet even with confusing sounds we have mastered the ABCs. Most likely, you were able to learn the alphabet because of repetition. Chances are you know a little tune whereby you can sing the ABCs on demand. The same strategies, plus some others, that worked when you were 5 years old can work for you now.

We are constantly taking in information, but the degree to which we remember or retrieve the information depends on several factors. Exposure or repetition is definitely a factor which affects our ability to remember an item. For instance, fill in the following:

"Meet George Jetson, his boy _____."

"That's the way we all became the _____ Bunch."

"It takes one to _____ one."

"I've been _____ on the railroad."

You have heard these phrases over and over until you automatically know the answer. Over-learning is an effective way to move information from your short-term memory to your long-term knowledge. Read and reread the information you are trying to memorize. Once you feel you have learned the material, then review it regularly to refresh your memory. Each time you review the material, it will take less and less time until you can anticipate words and phrases before you even read them. As you review material, recite it so you can see and hear the information. Writing and rewriting (more than once) will help you to retain information. Try to link new information with prior knowledge.

Use rhymes, acronyms, acrostics, and substitutions in familiar sayings or tunes. For instance, if you are trying to memorize the joints in the hands (MCP, PIP, DIP), you might memorize <u>My</u>

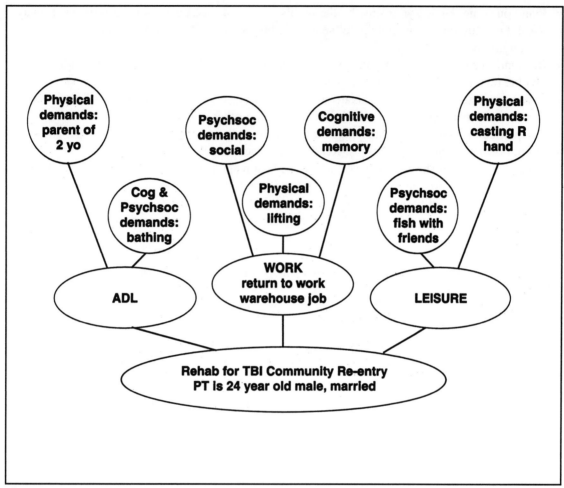

Figure 2-1. Occupational therapy mapping example.

Cousin Paul Put Ice Pieces Down Ida's Pants. Rearrange items in your list (unless they have to be remembered in a specific order) to make it easier to work with.

Test-taking strategies: Know the format of the test. It is easier to prepare when you know what the expectations are. For instance, on an essay test, you will have to retrieve information and do so in an orderly way. You will need to know pertinent vocabulary and how to use it appropriately. However, the reason you are reading this book is because of a certain little multiple choice test that is coming to a testing center near you. A multiple choice format is advantageous in that you need only to recognize the correct answer rather than generate it yourself. Still there are techniques that will enhance your chances of choosing the correct answer. The following are some tactics that will:

A. Help you to buy a new car
B. Help you lose 10 pounds
C. Get you a date with you-know-who
D. Help you succeed on the big test

The correct answer is D, the following test-taking strategies will help you succeed on the exam.

- Plan your time: Divide your time by the number of questions. Leave several minutes' leeway.
- Read the entire question: Anticipate the answer but do not be impulsive. Read each answer thoroughly before choosing.
- Respond to each question: If you leave it blank, it is definitely wrong. If you have absolutely no clue then make the best guess possible.
- If you are unsure of the answer: Narrow it down by eliminating the responses you know are incorrect. Sometimes you can get clues from reading other questions.
- Pay particular attention to qualifying words: Words such as *except, most, best, least,* and *not.*
- Do not over interpret the questions: Read them at face value.
- If you do not know the right answer: Make the best response possible and put a check by the question. If you have the time, return to the question to recheck. Do not waste time on the questions you do not know.
- If you must skip a question: Make absolutely sure that you skip the corresponding answer bubble. Again, you are better off answering all questions, and flag the ones you want to check later.
- A number two pencil means a number two pencil: Bring a minimum of three sharpened number two pencils with you on exam day.
- Continually check: Make sure the number of your question corresponds to the number on your answer sheet.
- Color in the bubbles nicely: Do not overdo it. Erase wrong answers completely.
- Trust your instincts: Do not second guess yourself. Be cautious about changing answers.
- Check the time: Check the clock or your watch occasionally to make sure you are on target.

READY TO STUDY

With supplies at hand, snacks in stock, and goal sheet pinned to your chest you are ready to get down and dirty. Before you sit down, you need to decide on a place for your intellectual experience (study environment). Consider the amount of noise, light, temperature, and physical comfort of your study area. In addition, will there be visual interference that will cause you to look up every few moments? Is your studying most effective morning, noon, or night? Make these decisions now to maximize your effectiveness.

Refer to your goal list to set expectations for each particular study session. Be aware that the first few minutes of your session are considered warm-up time that you will spend "shifting gears" and getting in the right mindset. Monitor your progress to check for fatigue and mind wandering. Evaluate your session afterwards to see if you were effective or if you need to change something for next time. Refer to the following study session evaluation checklist:

1. Did I have specific goals in mind as I sat down to study?
2. Were my expectations realistic?
3. Did I accomplish what I set out to do?
4. Was the time I set aside enough?
5. Did I implement specific study techniques based on my preferred learning style?
6. Was I distracted or tired?

TROUBLE SHOOTING

If your efforts are sincere but you are not getting the results you desire, refer to the following problem-solving solutions.

Trouble Shooting Solutions	
If:	*Try:*
You are sleepy	Physical activity, a break, a real nap, fresh air, a study partner, speaking aloud.
Your mind wanders	A new location, ear plugs, set smaller more obtainable goals, use manipulatives.
You are bored	Vary your routine, give yourself rewards, try 15 minutes on/15 minutes off, switch from reading to writing to speaking.
Too many interruptions	Take phone off hook/put answering machine on, put up a sign that says "Great mind at work—Please do not interrupt."
You are worried, overwhelmed	Break down tasks to even smaller chunks, see relaxation strategies.
You are forgetting previously learned material	Use clues to get information flowing, review less material more frequently, do not move to new concepts until old concepts are mastered, try learning through a different modality.
You are behind on your goals	Re-evaluate your time, double up on goals, refer to Chapter One for countdown calendar.

RELAXATION TECHNIQUES AND COPING SKILLS

As an occupational therapy student you have learned that relaxation techniques are effective for helping your patients to cope. Studying for the exam is a good time to use relaxation exercises yourself. The following exercises may be effective both before and during the exam.

Self talk: Ask yourself what is the worst thing that will happen if you do not study tonight or if you do not pass the test. Tell yourself that you can do this. You have done other hard things and can do this, too. You are great!

Review successes: Remind yourself of previous successes. You have made it this far. You have passed all your courses. You have passed other exams. You have completed a successful affiliation.

Take inventory: Do you know more than you did last year? Do you know more than you did last month? Have you studied/reviewed material recently?

Develop support systems: Let people know of your goals. Phone others to discuss your concerns. Be with people who will validate your self-worth.

Visualization: Picture yourself walking into the exam with confidence. Visualize yourself getting the results in the mail and scoring in the top 20%.

Daydream: Think about tanning on the beach, or skiing down a slope. Take a vacation in your mind.

Physical activity: Walking can clear your head and relax your muscles. Elevate your feet by lying on the floor and placing your feet on a chair for 10 minutes.

Deep breathing: Try deep cleansing breaths. Shut your eyes and slowly inhale through your nose. Hold the breath for 3 to 5 seconds and then exhale through your mouth. Repeat every time you feel stressed. If you are familiar with meditation techniques, try that after a few deep cleansing breaths.

SUMMARY

There is a satisfaction in knowing that one has done his or her best. The ideas presented in this chapter are suggestions to help you reach your goal of preparing, studying, and ultimately passing your examination. Preparing to study according to your strengths and weaknesses is an important part of studying effectively. Information regarding learning styles, organization, and specific study strategies is included in this chapter. It is important to develop the strategies that will be of most benefit to you. A study plan will ultimately help you save time and learn efficiently and effectively.

Chapter Three
Study Content Outlines

In this chapter you will find three outlines that cover the content topics on the exam. Each study outline covers content in one of three areas: physical management, mental health/cognitive management, and administration management. Special attention must be paid to the interaction of the physical and mental health management outlines. Expert occupational therapists know that pathology is not just physical or psychiatric. In addition, many other areas overlap such as frame of reference, impact of illness on function, and normal development. Be sure to review all the outlines for a more complete overview.

Each outline was developed by an expert OTR and is based on Uniform Terminology. If you are unfamiliar with Uniform Terminology, refer to Chapter One for information on how to get a copy. The outlines were developed using the knowledge statements from the Examination Content Outline by NBCOT. Information from other sources such as textbooks and AOTA's official papers were also used. As a student studying for the exam, you may want to use these outlines to develop your study plan or to double check your content after studying.

PHYSICAL MANAGEMENT CONTENT OUTLINE

I. Systems Review
   A. Structure and function of circulatory, respiratory, digestive, excretion, nervous

II. Tissue Types
   A. Connective tissue
      1. Tendon, ligaments, bone, cartilage

III. Joint Classification
   A. Diarthrodial/synovial
      1. Uniaxial, biaxial, triaxial
   B. Synarthrodial
   C. Amphiarthrodial

IV. Tissue Reaction to Disease and Injury
   A. Inflammation/edema
      1. Redness, pain, swelling, heat, decreased function
   B. Repair, healing stages

V. Causes of Disease and Disordered Function
   A. Etiology classifications
      1. Hereditary, congenital, traumatic, physical
      2. Chemical, infectious, inflammation, vascular, metabolic
      3. Nutritional, psychological, iatrogenic, idiopathic, tumors

VI. Frames of Reference
    A. Biomechanical
        1. Evaluation assesses physical limitations, ROM, strength, endurance
        2. Treatment to restore function
    B. Occupational performance
        1. Evaluation of performance components including sensorimotor, neuromuscular, motor, cognitive, psychosocial
        2. Treatment areas include activities of daily living, work, play/leisure
            a. Stage One: remediate performance components
            b. Stage Two: enabling activities
            c. Stage Three: purposeful activity
            d. Stage Four: community reintegration
    C. Rehabilitation
        1. Evaluation of abilities
        2. Treatment is restorative, acquisition of role performance
        3. Sensorimotor
        4. Evaluation of central nervous system dysfunction
        5. Treatment focus is sensory input leads to motor output, Rood, Bobath, Brunnstrom, PNF

VII. General Concerns of All Disorders
    A. Effects of inactivity on neuromuscular, musculoskeletal, digestive, respiratory, skin, cardiovascular, renal, psychosocial

VIII. Amputations
    A. Health concerns: etiology can be peripheral vascular disease, diabetes, trauma, COPD, and cardiac problems
    B. OT concerns: preprosthetic training, healing issues, cosmesis versus cosmetic, phantom pain, body image, prosthetic training, skin and stump care, donning and doffing, scar massage, adaptation, self-care, work, leisure, sexual adjustment

IX. Arthritis and Other Connective Tissue Disease
    A. Health concerns: disease process, systemic versus non-systemic, inflammatory versus noninflammatory, rapid versus insidious, exacerbation and remissions, secondary complications
    B. OT concerns: mobility and function, deformity, contractures, joint protection and body mechanics, adaptive equipment, energy conservation, work simplification, support group referral, rest, adapt home and work site, psychological support, sexual adjustment, family education

X. Burns
    A. Health concerns: classification, rule of nines, percent of total body surface area, first-degree superficial, second-degree partial thickness, third-degree full thickness, fourth-degree electrical, debridement, auto, full or split thickness grafts, shock, complications including pulmonary, metabolic, cardiac
    B. OT concerns: acute phase includes aseptic techniques, infection control, debridement;

rehabilitation phase includes hypertrophic scarring, heterotrophic bone ossification, and pressure gradient therapy; position of comfort may cause deformity; splints for oral, neck, elbow, axilla, hand, ankle; psychosocial adjustment, self-image, locus of control, community reentry

XI. Cancer
   A. Health concerns: improved diagnostic techniques including CT scan, PET scan, and MRI; prognosis varies by age, neurological status, tumor size, stage or grade, metastatic tumor from another site; treatments include surgery, radiation, and chemotherapy
   B. OT concerns: restorative, supportive, and palliative intervention, self-care, fatigue, ostomy care, mobility, pain, fear of recurrence, community involvement, vocational issues, hospice care, family education, home modification

XII. Cardiac Dysfunction
   A. Health concerns: medical history, shortness of breath, angina, MET levels, dyspnea, blood pressure, very light activity to 100 heart rate, avoid valsalva maneuver, arrhythmia
   B. OT concerns: lifestyle, avocational interests, stress, adjustment to limitations, energy conservation, work simplification, graded exercise routine, psychosocial adjustment, family education, safety, role adjustments

XIII. Cerebral Palsy
   A. Health concerns: prenatal, perinatal, postnatal, tone is mixed, spastic or dystonia, athetoid, ataxia, praxis, oral motor and feeding problems, dysarthria, mental retardation possible
   B. OT concerns: sensory processing, developmental delays, primitive reflex activity, bilateral integration, ADLs, early intervention, school intervention and inclusion, play, family support and education, wheelchair positioning, splinting, adaptive equipment, home modifications

XIV. Cerebral Vascular Accident
   A. Health concerns: thrombus, embolus, aneurysm, hemorrhage, TIA, anoxia, middle cerebral artery, lesion side has contralateral hemiplegia, reflex sympathetic dystrophy
   B. OT concerns: Left CVA may include right hemiplegia or hemiparesis, apraxia, hemianopsia, impaired sequencing skills, be slow or cautious and show receptive, expressive, or global aphasia. Right CVA may include left hemiplegia or hemiparesis, hemianopsia, visual spatial deficits, left in attention, position in space problems, and denial of illness. All CVAs may show sensory loss, synergy, tone, decreased function in ADLs, work, or leisure. Changed self-image, isolation, home modification, driver training, adaptive equipment, safety, family education.

XV. Chronic Pain Conditions
   A. Health concerns: noscioceptive or persistent pain, abusing pain medication
   B. OT concerns: maladaptive responses, depression, withdrawal from roles, conditioning exercises, work hardening, stress reduction, leisure activities, supportive environment, positive self-talk, visualization, self-hypnosis, imagery, nutrition, family support

XVI. Guillain-Barré and Motor Unit Diseases
   A. Health concerns: demyelination, spinal nerve roots, peripheral nerves
   B. OT concerns: sensory loss, muscle atrophy, contractures, fatigue, endurance, oral motor function, respiratory problems, decreased trunk control, fine and gross motor coordination, ataxia, pain, psychosocial adjustments, home modifications, ADLs, work and leisure, incomplete recovery

XVII. Hand Injuries
   A. Health concerns: joint injuries and deformities; tendon injuries; nerve compression and injuries in median, radial, or ulnar nerves; muscle imbalance; atrophy or weakness
   B. OT concerns: loss of sensation, decreased functional grasp and pinch, sensory discrimination, fine motor skills, loss of function in ADL, work, and leisure

XVIII. Head Injuries
   A. Health concerns: orthopedic such as fractures, heterotopic ossification, neurological, coupe and countercoupe, cerebral contusions, frontal and temporal lobe involvement common, cranial nerves, coma and altered level of consciousness, amnesia, seizures, hydrocephalus
   B. OT concerns: sensory loss, visual perceptual and vision changes, cognitive executive function, motoric loss, behavioral changes, aphasia, dysphagia, self-care, work productivity, leisure, adaptive equipment, splints, driver training, family education, safety in motor, cognitive, and behavior

XIX. Hip Fracture
   A. Health concerns: total hip arthroplasty, arthrodesis, total hip articular replacement with internal eccentric shells, restricted mobility, pain, age as an issue
   B. OT concerns: mobility, independence, fear of reinjury, adaptive equipment, loss of roles, home modification, endurance, adaptive equipment

XX. Multiple Sclerosis and Other Degenerative Diseases
   A. Health concerns: CNS disorder, exacerbation and remission, unpredictable process
   B. OT concerns: muscle weakness, incoordination, tremors, sensory loss, pain, proprioception loss, visual disturbances including diplopia, dysarthria, bladder problems, psychological adjustment including depression and euphoria, cognitive involvement, support group referral, home and work site adaptations, safety issues, adaptive equipment, family education, ongoing driving evaluation

XXI. Muscular Dystrophy
   A. Health concerns: genetic disorder, major progressive muscle weakness, atrophy of limbs and trunk, pulmonary problems, Gower's sign, lordosis, scoliosis, fat replaces muscle, cardiac complications, scapula winging
   B. OT concerns: prevent contractures, splinting, adaptive equipment, muscle imbalance, ADLs, school intervention and inclusion, play, gait disturbances, mild cognitive problems, maintain function, family support and education, wheelchair positioning, home modifications

XXII. Spinal Cord Injuries
    A. Health concerns: orthopedic, neurological, cardiopulmonary, autonomic dysreflexia, postural hypotension, deceased temperature regulation
    B. OT concerns: sensory loss, splints, body image, bowel and bladder function, strengthening, personal relationships, sexual readjustment, self-care, work productivity, leisure, home modification, adaptive equipment, driver education, family education

XXIII. Spina Bifida
    A. Health concerns: failure of fusion, neural arches, meningocele, open or closed sac, surgery, infection, hydrocephalus
    B. OT concerns: gross motor and developmental disturbances, self-care, school intervention and inclusion, adaptive equipment, wheelchair positioning, home modifications, family support and education

MENTAL HEALTH/COGNITIVE MANAGEMENT CONTENT OUTLINE

I. Normal Development
    A. Life cycle theory
        1. Piaget, Gesell, Sullivan, Kohlberg, Freud, Erikson
        2. Stages, landmarks, crisis points, cultural impact
    B. Developmental theory
        1. Physical, cognitive, and emotional milestones from birth to death

II. Frames of Reference
    A. Behavioral
        1. Evaluation is of adaptive or maladaptive behaviors
        2. Treatment based on classical and operant conditioning. Techniques such as shaping, chaining, token economy, and biofeedback are used to reinforce desired behavior.
    B. Cognitive behavioral
        1. Evaluation of self-regulation and self-control
        2. Treatment involves reinforcement, modeling, and observation; develop insight and understanding; modify how person thinks
    C. Cognitive disability
        1. Evaluation is on assessing cognitive functioning level
        2. Treatment is based on brain pathology; match activities to cognitive level by changing activity not person; function exists when person is capable of meeting routine task demands
    D. Developmental
        1. Evaluation is of specific stages that are progressive and hierarchical
        2. Treatment addresses developmental themes, groups are based on different levels, drive toward mastery, skills must be learned in sequence of normal development
    E. Model of human occupation
        1. Evaluation looks at volition, habituation, and performance
        2. Treatment based on human as an open system that can change through interaction with the environment, competency is based on ability to perform daily tasks, directive groups

F. Psychodynamic
   1. Evaluation of unconscious conflict; aspects of personality, id, ego, superego
   2. Treatment integrates wants, needs, and drives in conscious awareness, object relations, transference and counter transference, defenses, therapeutic sense of self
G. Sensory integration
   1. Evaluation is of brain's ability to filter, organize, and integrate sensory information; look for mature adaptive responses
   2. Treatment is based on neuroscience, neuropsychology, and neurophysiology; vestibular, tactile, and proprioceptive input impacts postural control, body schema, bonding, coordination, language, perception, emotions and is base for visual and auditory functions, related to learning disabilities in children, process is developmental
H. Therapeutic process
   1. Patient/therapist relationship
      a. Counseling skills, ethics, confidentiality
   2. Environment
      a. Structure versus unstructured, hospital, community milieu, and group homes
   3. Role of occupational therapy on a multidisciplinary team
      a. Role of other members on treatment team

III. Alcohol and Other Substance Abuse
   A. Health concerns: difference between abuse and dependency, effects on CNS, etiology includes genetic, neurochemical, and environmental factors, slippage is common
   B. OT concerns: assess suicidal potential; vocational, social, and leisure components mostly impacted; dual diagnosis with another mental health disability; transference and counter transference are often magnified

IV. Alzheimer and Other Dementia Disorders
   A. Health concerns: etiology includes neurochemical, environmental, viral, trauma, genetic, and substance abuse
   B. OT concerns: awareness, orientation, organization, attention, problem solving, decision making, reasoning, insight, judgment, functional adaptation, supervision needed, remedial techniques, safety, perceptual problems may not be apparent at first, family education and support

V. Anxiety Disorders
   A. Health concerns: anxiety can be mild to severe, antianxiety medication helpful, PTSD always stems from a trauma
   B. OT concerns: assess suicidal potential, avoidance behaviors shown, occupational and social functioning impaired, behavioral techniques such as relaxation, desensitization, and imagery effective

VI. Attention Deficit Disorder and ADHD
   A. Health concerns: etiology may be neurological in combination with environmental factors, medication
   B. OT concerns: low stimulation environment, mastery of developmental skills, self-regulation, self-advocacy skills, family education, inclusion in school

VII. Bipolar Disorder, Depression, and Other Affective Disorders
  A. Health concerns: familial patterns are common, depression is most common of all psychiatric disorders, medication such as an antidepressant and lithium manage symptoms
  B. OT concerns: assess suicidal potential, use precautions due to decreased judgment, may affect all performance areas especially social, activities need to be gratifying

VIII. Eating Disorders
  A. Health concerns: includes anorexia nervosa and bulimia, medical management of weight, etiology usually includes family dysfunction, nutritional needs, biological changes, may be chronic and lifetime disease
  B. OT concerns: asssess suicidal potential; personality traits include decreased self-esteem, perfectionism, and need for control; food is major focus, develop interest in activities; social skills and leisure are critical areas

IX. Mental Retardation
  A. Health concerns: Down syndrome or other genetic causes, other disabilities such as seizures or physical issues, medications
  B. OT concerns: sensory and neurodevelopmental approaches to minimize physical problems and encourage developmental skills, social skills training, vocational training, family support, inclusion, ADL and leisure education, sexual education

X. Learning Disabilities
  A. Health concerns: etiology may be neurological
  B. OT concerns: appropriate learning, mastery of developmental skills, self-advocacy skills, family education, accommodations and inclusion in the classroom

XI. Personality Disorders
  A. Health concerns: lifelong patterns, inaccurate perception of self and others
  B. OT concerns: assess suicidal potential, poor personal values and goals, relationship problems, individual versus group treatment depends on disorder, transference and countertransference, vocational, social, and leisure are mostly affected

XII. Schizophrenia and Other Psychotic Disorders
  A. Health concerns: thought disorder including hallucinations and delusions, positive versus negative symptoms, often chronic in nature, medication side effects such as tardive dyskinesia and extrapyramidal symptoms
  B. OT concerns: assess suicidal potential, all performance areas affected, do not challenge psychotic thinking, address sensorimotor and cognitive disabilities, behavioral techniques, medication regime

XIII. Occupational Therapy Groups
  A. Theory
    1. Fidler's task oriented, Mosey and Llorens' developmental, Allen's cognitive levels, Kaplan's directive, Ross' structured five stage
  B. Group or individual treatment topics examples by performance components
    1. Sensorimotor
      a. Sensory integration and movement groups

2. Cognitive
   a. Task and project groups
3. Psychosocial
   a. Creative and projective arts groups
C. Group or individual treatment topic examples by performance areas
   1. Activities of daily living
      a. Social skills, sexual expression, grooming, time management, dressing, cooking
   2. Work and productive activities
      a. Prevocational, work exploration, work hardening, parenting, retirement, home making, sensory integration, play, coping skills, assertiveness
   3. Play or leisure.
      a. Play, dance, music, arts and crafts, leisure exploration

ADMINISTRATION MANAGEMENT CONTENT OUTLINE

I. Program Development
   A. Needs assessment
      1. Focus group, demographics, key informants, survey, questionnaire
   B. Program planning
      1. Philosophy, mission statement, goals, and objectives
   C. Treatment
      1. Referral, screening, assessment, intervention plan, intervention including direct and consulting, transition services, discontinuation
   D. Program evaluation

II. Program Management
   A. Management by objectives (MBO), organizational policies including ADA and OBRA, accreditation requirements including JCAHO, CARF, and state requirements
   B. Documentation
      1. Objective versus subjective, identify patient's strengths and weaknesses
      2. Requirements, format including SOAP, POMR, and narrative
   C. Reimbursement
      1. DRGs, Medicare part A, Medicare part B, CHAMPUS, private third party payers including nonprofit and for profit, HMOs, worker's compensation
   D. Quality assurance and continuous quality improvement
   E. Budget and financial aspects
      1. Supplies and equipment, direct versus indirect, capital expenses, fixed versus variable expenses
   F. OT promotion
   G. Ethics
      1. Reporting violations
   H. Standards of practice
   I. Safety standards
      1. Universal precautions, environmental health, incident reports
   J. Continuing education
      1. Update theories and techniques

K. Patient rights
  1. Confidentiality, refuse treatment
L. Research
  1. Benefits
M. AOTA, AOTF, NBCOT

III. Personnel Management
  A. OT personnel and credentialing OTR, COTA, OT aide
  B. Productivity
    1. Measurement methods and performance appraisals
  C. Supervision
  D. Staff retention
  E. Functions of an OT
    1. Uniform Terminology, role delineation of OTR and COTA
    2. Collaboration of the OTR and COTA
  F. Malpractice and liability

Chapter Four
Fieldwork Experience as a Study Guide

ROLE OF FIELDWORK

The purpose of fieldwork is to integrate classroom study with clinical practice and develop clinical reasoning skills. To help you use your fieldwork experience to study for the exam, you must first understand some of the policies established by AOTA.

Fieldwork in an accredited OTR school is divided into two types: Level I and Level II. Level I fieldwork is experienced during your studies, usually done part-time during the academic year. Level II is typically full-time, after you have completed your studies. Of course, due to the shortages of fieldwork sites, your school may have provided you with a creative, nontraditional Level II fieldwork. Although these fieldwork experiences are different from what has been traditional in the past, it is our experience that these students do equally well on the exam.

Much of what you know as an occupational therapy student was developed and refined during your fieldwork experiences. This section of the book is designed to help you review your fieldwork experience. We have provided opportunities to reflect on your areas of accomplishment and those that need further review before you take the exam. Begin by identifying all of your fieldwork sites using the example below.

Sample Fieldwork Review			
Fieldwork Sites	*Level I*	*Level II*	*On My Own*
St. Mary's Hospital	Observed hand tx		Observed peds
Community Mental Health Center		Community skills assessments	
Summer Program for Special Kids			Helped OTR run SI groups

Use the following table to identify your fieldwork experiences. Fill in each square with a brief summary of what you did at each fieldwork site. Include Levels I and II fieldwork and any additional experiences you have had working with an OTR.

Fieldwork Review			
Fieldwork Sites	*Level I*	*Level II*	*On My Own*

Now that you have reviewed your fieldwork experiences, it is time to look at the variety of consumers you have worked with. Below is a table of diagnostic categories that many OTRs work with. It is not expected that you have had experiences in all these areas. On the contrary, students who focused their experiences in limited areas developed clinical reasoning more easily. This table is designed to point out which areas you are accomplished in and which areas you may need to review before the exam. Use a check mark to indicate your assessment of your fieldwork experience. Blank spaces are provided at the end of the table to add other diagnostic categories.

Fieldwork Diagnosis Review				
Diagnosis	*No Experience*	*Observation Experience*	*Some Experience*	*A Lot of Experience*
AIDS				
Amputation				
Arthritis				
Bipolar disorder				
Burns				
Cancer				
Cardiac disease				
Cerebral palsy				
Child/elder abuse				
CVA				
Dementia				
Depression				
Drug/alcohol abuse				
Eating disorders				
Failure to thrive				
Hand/arm conditions				
Head injuries				
Kidney disease				
Learning disabilities				
Mental retardation				
Multiple sclerosis				
Muscular dystrophy				
Orthopedic conditions				

Personality disorders				
Schizophrenia				
SI dysfunction				
Spina bifida				
Spinal cord injuries				

After you have completed a review of your fieldwork experiences, it is time to make an assessment of the areas you need to review before the exam. Fieldwork was never intended to provide you with a view of all occupational therapy practice. It would be expected that many of your check marks on the fieldwork diagnosis review table would be in the "no experience" column.

Setting studying priorities for the exam should begin in the "no experience" and "observation experience" columns. Even with that as a starting place, you may feel like it is too much to manage at once. Use the study priorities chart to set your study priorities.

Study Priorities			
Diagnosis	*Top Priority*	*Second Priority*	*No Need to Study*
AIDS			
Amputation			
Arthritis			
Bipolar disorder			
Burns			
Cancer			
Cardiac disease			
Cerebral palsy			
Child/elder abuse			
CVA			
Dementia			
Depression			
Drug/alcohol abuse			
Eating disorders			
Failure to thrive			
Hand/arm conditions			
Head injuries			
Kidney disease			
Learning disabilities			
Mental retardation			

Multiple sclerosis			
Muscular dystrophy			
Orthopedic conditions			
Personality disorders			
Schizophrenia			
SI dysfunction			
Spina bifida			
Spinal cord injuries			

Now that you have set your topic priorities, consider the amount of time available before the exam and what time you have outside of your current life responsibilities to study. Review Chapter Two and incorporate your priorities in your study plan. Next review the chapters that outline physical, mental health/cognitive, and administration management content earlier in this book.

When working on the study questions in the next section, you may find it helpful to recall some of your patients from your affiliations to problem solve the answer to a question. You can organize your study review notes based on classic symptoms versus clinical symptoms you saw on your affiliations. This will allow you to think through a question on the exam with a story visualization of what the patient would look like. Review the following example and then fill out your own table.

Sample Classic versus Clinical Pictures During Fieldwork			
Diagnosis	*Patient's First Name*	*Classic Symptoms*	*Clinical Symptoms Seen on Fieldwork*
CVA-left cortex	Samuel	expressive aphasia	mild
		receptive aphasia	not present
		right side weakness	yes
		spaticity	yes, required splint
Schizophrenia	Anna	withdrawn	no
		flat affect	blunted but not flat
		hallucinations	heard voices
		delusions	no
		poor hygiene	good with reminder

Use the following table to outline your own patient stories. Fill in the spaces with the classic symptoms based on your class notes and textbooks. Picture the patient in your mind and fill in the clinical symptoms you saw during your fieldwork.

This exercise will help you answer exam questions using the clinical reasoning skills you developed during fieldwork. When faced with a question such as developing a treatment activity for a person with schizophrenia or a CVA, picture your patient trying each of the available answers. This might help you eliminate wrong answers and zero in on the correct answer.

Classic versus Clinical Pictures During Fieldwork			
Diagnosis	*Patient's First Name*	*Classic Symptoms*	*Clinical Symptoms Seen on Fieldwork*

SUMMARY

Reviewing your fieldwork experiences will help you recognize both accomplishments and areas that need further study. Examining each different diagnosis that you saw during both Level I and Level II fieldwork will help you to prioritize studying for the exam. Visualizing patient stories in your mind may help you eliminate wrong answers on the exam and remember correct ones.

SECTION III
Study Questions

Look in
dew book

Chapter Five
Study Questions

GETTING DOWN TO BUSINESS

The NBCOT exam has a total of 200 questions and a time limit of 4 hours. This means that you need to answer 50 questions per hour. To help you get ready for the NBCOT exam, we have designed our study questions to simulate some of the factors you will notice when you take the real exam. First, we have divided our 450 study questions into 50-question sections. Although our study questions are different from the real exam questions, you can use them to pace yourself when studying. If you are working on pacing yourself, you should try to complete one section per hour. Consider using a timer or stopwatch. Second, we have mixed the topics of our study questions like the NBCOT exam. This means that you might answer a question on CVA followed by a question on group process. Lastly, we have provided you with bubble sheets (Appendix D) to put your answers on. Simply tear out a blank answer sheet for each section of study questions you complete. We recommend that you use a number two pencil to mark your answers on the bubble sheet so that you get a feel for how many sharp pencils you will need for exam day. Answers and explanations for all the questions are available in Chapter Six.

Remember to read each study question carefully. Pay attention to detail words such as *except, most, best, least,* and *not.* The exam questions, as well as our study questions, are not trick questions. If you do not understand the question the first time you read it, read it again slowly.

STUDY QUESTIONS

Section One

1. The C6 client you are working with complains of dizziness and nausea and seems to be losing consciousness as you bring him to standing in the standing table. Your best course of action is:
   A. Wait, the symptoms should pass as tolerance increases
   B. Bring him down to the wheelchair again
   C. Call for his nurse
   D. Bring him down to the wheelchair and then immediately recline him

2. A performance skill for a client in a low back pain program would be:
   A. Muscle strength
   B. Work tolerance
   C. Cognitive functioning
   D. Lifting tolerance

3. Choose the item that does *not* describe normal developmental expectations for an 8-year-old:
   A. Project level play is preferred
   B. Deductive reasoning is possible
   C. Playing dress up is a favored activity
   D. Has the ability to perceive and organize information

4. To be reimbursed under Medicare Part B, outpatient occupational therapy services must do all of the following *except*:
   A. Meet conditions set forth in coverage guidelines
   B. Services must be furnished under a written plan
   C. A physician must certify need for treatment
   D. The OTR must be hospital affiliated

5. Inflammation of the common extensor origin of the forearm extensor musculature may result in:
   A. Gamekeeper's thumb
   B. Golfer's elbow
   C. Tennis elbow
   D. Pitcher's shoulder

6. An OTR using the psychoanalytic frame of reference suggests kneading dough to make bread as an activity for a nonverbal and angry patient. The OTR is basing her activity choice on which of the following concepts?
   A. Acting out
   B. Sublimation
   C. Identification
   D. Regression

7. Uniform Terminology delineates and defines occupational therapy direct services. Which is *not* true of Uniform Terminology?
   A. It provides a fee structure, flexible for use in different programs
   B. It is used by AOTA in many official documents
   C. It provides a base of consistent terminology
   D. It is updated periodically in accordance with current theory and practice

8. Entry-level COTAs are allowed to perform occupational therapy if supervised by:
   A. A nursing director
   B. A physician
   C. Another COTA who has experience
   D. An OTR

9. Degenerative disorders commonly associated with depression, dementia, and psychosis include all of the following *except*:
   A. Parkinson's disease
   B. Huntington's disease
   C. Wilson's disease
   D. Connective tissue disease

10. Which ligament limits vertebral column extension?
    A. Posterior longitudinal ligament
    B. Ligamentum flavum
    C. Supraspinatus
    D. Anterior longitudinal ligament

11. In a 6-month-old child, symptoms such as abnormal muscle tone, delayed or exaggerated reflexes, postural abnormalities, and delayed motor development are signs of:
    A. Nothing to worry about, some 6-month-old children are like that
    B. Autism
    C. Mental retardation
    D. Cerebral palsy

12. Emotional flight in an emergency situation is dominated by which nervous system?
    A. Peripheral nervous system
    B. Sympathetic nervous system
    C. Parasympathetic nervous system
    D. Central nervous system

13. Direct occupational therapy services include:
    A. The OTR as consultant
    B. A focus on wellness and prevention
    C. A hands-on, face-to-face relationship between the client and the therapist
    D. The OTR as fieldwork supervisor

14. A patient who experiences abrupt changes and swings in emotional tone despite what is occurring in his or her external environment is *best* described as:
    A. Labile
    B. Anhedonia
    C. Inappropriate
    D. Euphoric

15. All of the following are clinical symptoms of spasticity *except*:
    A. A stretch reflex
    B. Clonus
    C. Atrophy
    D. Hyperactive tendon tap

16. A self-employed OTR does contract work in several nursing homes. Who is responsible for malpractice and liability insurance?
    A. Each nursing home covers the OTR while he or she is working at the facility
    B. AOTA covers the OTR
    C. The state department of nursing home licensure covers the OTR
    D. Each OTR must carry individual coverage

17. Documentation of OT services to a patient should include all of the following *except*:
    A. The patient's response to treatment
    B. The treatment techniques used
    C. The patient's bill balance
    D. A plan for future treatment

18. Your client is a 70-year-old male who lived alone just prior to having a total hip replacement. In order to manage his self-care, the *best* equipment he will need is:
    A. A tea cart with wheels for the kitchen
    B. Dressing stick, sock aid, longhandled shoe horn, bath sponge, and reacher
    C. Tub seat adjusted to his tub at home
    D. Commode for bedside

19. A quadriplegic patient at the C5 level would have little or no wrist and finger function. The goal of OT would be to enhance wrist extension and tenodesis grasp. How can this *best* be done?
    A. Range finger flexion with wrist flexed
    B. Range finger extension with wrist extended
    C. Range finger flexion with wrist fully extended, finger extension with wrist fully flexed
    D. Makes no difference

20. Licensure for OTRs is granted by:
    A. AOTA
    B. NBCOT
    C. A state agency
    D. Both NBCOT and a state agency

21. Many health care programs use management by objective (MBO) plans for the administration of their programs. A MBO plan includes:
    A. A problem-oriented medical record
    B. Overall objective, derived goals, key participants
    C. Subjective, objective, assessment, plan
    D. Indicators, monitors, quality improvement

22. Which of the following behavioral techniques would be *most* appropriate to use with a patient who has agoraphobia?
    A. Habilitation
    B. Extinction
    C. Systematic desensitization
    D. Token economy

23. The Brunnstrom approach to the treatment of hemiplegia incorporates the use of synergy action. The components of the flexor synergy for the shoulder include:
    A. Scapular adduction, depression, shoulder adduction, and internal rotation
    B. Scapular adduction, elevation, shoulder abduction, and external rotation
    C. Scapular abduction, protraction, shoulder adduction, and internal rotation
    D. Scapular abduction, retraction, shoulder abduction

24. The components for the flexor synergy of the elbow and forearm include:
    A. Elbow extension and forearm supination
    B. Elbow flexion and forearm supination
    C. Elbow extension and forearm neutral
    D. Elbow extension and forearm pronation

25. Outpatient occupational therapy services are covered under Medicare Part B when:
    A. No OT is available at a local hospital
    B. Part of an office visit to a physician
    C. Not related to a specific condition
    D. Part A is used up

26. A 60-year-old female client with a history of multiple sclerosis is managed at home with specific adaptations to facilitate function. The patient's family has provided significant care in the area of self-care. You are treating the patient in home care and have noticed she is more withdrawn and recently complained of difficulty swallowing. What is the *best* intervention?
    A. Supportive questioning and explore respite care
    B. Mention to the family your concern
    C. Keep a good log of the patient's responses in therapy
    D. Attribute mood changes and minor problems to nature of the chronic disease

27. The term that describes principles of occupational therapy practice for individual patients, including guidelines for determining function/dysfunction, motivation, and the change process, is called:
    A. Paradigm
    B. Model
    C. Frame of reference
    D. Therapeutic use of self

28. A lesion in the cerebellum may cause which type of tone?
    A. Rigidity
    B. Hypertonia
    C. Hypotonia
    D. Spasticity

29. Which piece of adaptive equipment is *most* appropriate for a patient with a total knee replacement?
    A. Longhandled shoe horn
    B. Reacher
    C. Sock aid
    D. None of the above

30. Spinal nerves are formed by joining dorsal and ventral roots. They are composed of a mixture of motor, sensory, and autonomic fibers. The ventral root carries which type of information?
    A. Sensory/afferent
    B. Sensory/efferent
    C. Motor/afferent
    D. Motor/efferent

31. The incidence of depression among institutionalized elderly is more prevalent than among their peers living independently in the community. Which of the following statements is the greatest predictor for depression within this long-term elderly population?
    A. Loss of ability to perform ADLs
    B. Late onset of clinical depression
    C. Cognitive impairment
    D. Family history of depression

Use the following to answer questions 32 through 36: As more occupational therapists work in cardiac rehabilitation including outpatient or community settings, the understanding of certain concepts is key to good care delivery. For example, the term "MET" is used in exercise physiology. One MET is equal to 3.5 ml oxygen/kg. This describes the energy required for the average person at rest, such as sitting quietly.

32. On average, self-care activities are at what MET level?
    A. 1
    B. 3
    C. 5
    D. 7

33. Signs of activity-induced cardiovascular dysfunction include all of the following *except*:
    A. Fever
    B. Dyspnea
    C. Altered mental status
    D. Fatigue

34. A cardiac patient in phase 1 in rehabilitation can begin exercise when this occurs:
    A. Generally, 4 days after admission to the hospital
    B. Depression lifts
    C. Free of chest pain
    D. Decrease in anxiety

35. At what point in cardiac rehabilitation does education on diet, stress, medication, and exercise begin?
    A. Phase 1
    B. Phase 2
    C. Phase 3
    D. At discharge

36. The occupational therapist in a cardiac rehabilitation program would consider which goal most valuable in the education phase of the patient?
    A. Vocational modification
    B. Energy conservation
    C. Sexual counseling
    D. Relaxation techniques

37. Which reflex is responsible for maintaining normal muscle tone or resistance to movement?
    A. Phasic/dynamic reflex
    B. Static/tonic stretch reflex
    C. Inverse stretch reflex
    D. Withdrawal/flexor reflex

38. According to the National Institute of Mental Health, which of the following statements about suicide is *false*?
    A. More men than women die by suicide, a ratio of 4:1
    B. Suicide by firearms is the most common method for both men and women
    C. The highest suicide rates are for persons over 65 years of age
    D. Inquiring about suicidal thoughts will implant ideas in people

39. Health care professionals who experience emotional exhaustion, diminished positive feelings toward others, and reduced personal accomplishment may be experiencing what syndrome?
    A. Clinical depression
    B. Dysthymia
    C. Burnout
    D. Stress reaction

40. The OT clinic must have available MSDS (material safety data sheets) on all of the following *except*:
    A. White out
    B. Theraputty
    C. Soaps
    D. Personal items

41. Often COTAs and OTRs work together on the treatment of a particular client. Which is the *best* way to document supervision of the treatment and COTA by the OTR?
    A. The OTR cosigns the treatment notes in the medical record
    B. The OTR keeps a supervision log book when discussing treatment with the COTA
    C. No special documentation is needed because billing is the same for COTAs and OTRs
    D. A third party, such as the OT supervisor, documents the collaboration

42. Scapulohumeral rhythm must be taken into account when ranging a shoulder. What is the ratio of scapulohumeral rhythm?
    A. 1:2 scapula:humerus
    B. 2:1 scapula:humerus
    C. 1:4 scapula:humerus
    D. 4:1 scapula:humerus

43. What pediatric diagnosis is characterized by loss of hand skills developed and abnormal hand movements such as hand wringing and hand washing?
    A. Childhood disintegrative disorder
    B. Childhood schizophrenia
    C. Autism
    D. Rett's syndrome

44. What are signs of sensory integrative dysfunction?
    A. Oversensitivity to sound, movement, touch, or visual input
    B. Impulsive, lack of self-control, distraction
    C. Poor self-concept, social problems
    D. All of the above

45. Which is *false* concerning NDT theory?
    A. Abnormal muscle tone affects muscles but not feeding, speech, or perception
    B. The central nervous system is damaged resulting in abnormal movements
    C. Change in motor patterns results from the individual feeling more normal movements
    D. An interdisciplinary effort achieves the optimal gains for the individual

46. All of the following techniques are available to the occupational therapist using a cognitive behavioral approach *except*:
    A. Free association
    B. Graded task assignments
    C. Bibliotherapy
    D. Role modeling

47. An activity group in which the client learns group interaction skills through sequential, stage-specific skills is called?
    A. Developmental group
    B. Task-oriented group
    C. Evaluation group
    D. Instrumental group

48. In general, which type of muscle structure provides the greatest ROM?
    A. Fusiform/strap
    B. Spiral
    C. Multipennate
    D. Unipennate

49. According to Yalom, which type of leadership style is most useful in the acute, inpatient therapy group?
    A. Advisory
    B. Facilitative
    C. Directive
    D. Democratic

50. The occupational therapist has been asked to evaluate a feeding program for a 65-year-old woman with hemiplegia. The patient spilled food because of the inability to adjust her movement when getting food to the mouth. The *most* likely neurobehavioral impairment is:
    A. Ideational apraxia
    B. Motor apraxia
    C. Unilateral body neglect
    D. Perseveration

Section Two

1. Can occupational therapy services be started for a Medicare patient at home?
   A. Only if physical therapy, nursing, or speech is also servicing the patient
   B. Yes, even if OT is alone
   C. Only if two physicians order OT
   D. Yes, if DRGs are still available

2. During an occupational therapy task group, the OTR asks a patient to check out his self-perception with others in the group. This thinking process is called:
   A. Autistic thinking
   B. Reality testing
   C. Magical thinking
   D. Illogical thinking

3. Dysdiadochokinesia is a neurological disorder defined as:
   A. A motor problem seen as overshooting or past pointing
   B. A motor problem where muscles are weak and tire easily
   C. The impaired ability for rapid, repeated alternating movements
   D. Slow, twisting movements

4. The client you are treating is a 60-year-old female with a right CVA. She shows left hemiplegia, severe left homonymous hemianopsia, and left neglect. The *best* approach to facilitate acknowledgment of the left spatial and visual field is:
   A. Remind client to look to the left
   B. Ask family to remind client to look to the left
   C. Ask nursing to remind client to look to the left
   D. Arrange client's environment so it encourages the client to look to the left

5. A hemiplegic patient with shoulder subluxation is *best* treated by:
   A. Wearing of sling for 24 hours a day
   B. Only wearing a sling during gait training
   C. Proper positioning while in bed and in wheelchair
   D. A lap board while in wheelchair

6. What type of prehension is used to pick up small objects such as pins, nails, or buttons?
   A. Palmar prehension, palmar tripod, or three jaw chuck
   B. Lateral prehension
   C. Hook grasp
   D. Fingertip prehension

7. When measuring for a wheelchair, what consideration should be made for the seat?
   A. None, seat is standard, no measurements are needed
   B. If doorways in patient's home are narrow, wheelchair seat must be narrow
   C. Seat should be 4 inches wider than patient's widest point across hips or thighs so he or she can move around easier
   D. Seat should be 2 inches wider than patient's widest point across hips or thighs. If braces are worn, width should be increased

8. What fine motor activity is *best* for a 6-year-old child with attention deficit disorder?
   A. Dot-to-dot coloring
   B. Musical instrument such as the piano
   C. Handling a deck of cards
   D. Mazes

9. While performing PROM on your client, you notice spasticity during elbow flexion. Following the spasitcity, you notice a sudden relaxation and letting go of tone and full range is achieved. This is called:
   A. Claspknife phenomenon
   B. Clonus
   C. Rigidity
   D. Dystonia

10. A confused head injured patient may ask a lot of questions, often repeating the same question over and over. What is the *best* activity for this patient?
    A. Nothing, the patient is too agitated
    B. Socializing with other patients
    C. Looking at his or her memory book
    D. Playing cards

11. The difference between high technology and low technology is:
    A. Cost
    B. Design
    C. Electronics
    D. Patient diagnosis

12. Which of the following terms describes symptoms caused by abstinence from a substance which the patient has taken over a period of time?
    A. Addiction
    B. Intoxication
    C. Withdrawal
    D. Abuse

13. While assessing the mental status of a patient, the OTR could observe which of the following without asking a direct question?
    A. If the patient can subtract 7 from 100 to measure visuospatial ability
    B. If the patient's affect can be described as normal, flat, blunted, constricted
    C. If the patient has visual hallucinations showing a disturbance in thought process
    D. The patient's mood

14. Residents of a nursing home are often lifetime members of the nursing home community. An OTR working in a nursing home must therefore address a resident's needs as if it is his or her home. What activity *best* facilitates fine motor coordination and community development?
    A. Sponsor a float in a community parade, residents can watch
    B. Develop a facility choir and perform for everyone while holding choir music
    C. Make a quilt and raffle it off to purchase something for the facility
    D. Build birdhouses and install them outside the windows of bedfast residents

15. When working in an activity group with a patient who has AIDS, the occupational therapist should:
   A. Always wear latex gloves
   B. Wash hands before and after treatment
   C. Avoid touching the patient
   D. Always wear a face mask

16. Which early childhood disease is progressive, fatal, and due to fatty fibrous infiltration of muscles?
   A. Post-polio syndrome
   B. Muscular dystrophy
   C. Parkinson's disease
   D. Multiple sclerosis

17. Premature infants usually have mothers who have low socioeconomic status, lack of prenatal care, and poor nutrition. A premature infant is any infant born before:
   A. 37 weeks
   B. 39 weeks
   C. 41 weeks
   D. 43 weeks

18. Vestibular stimulation can be used to increase muscle tone in both adults and children. Always watch the patient for emotional reactions. Spinning should *not* be done with what type of person?
   A. Persons over the age of 50
   B. Persons with poor ROM
   C. Persons prone to seizures
   D. Persons who are 6 feet or over in height

19. Spina bifida is a disorder characterized by failure of the vertebral column to close. Children may have a shunt placed in their head. All of the following are warning signs of a malfunctioning shunt *except*:
   A. Irritability and fussiness
   B. Vomiting
   C. Headache
   D. Wide open eyes, iris is totally visible

20. An upper motor neuron lesion may occur in all of the following *except*:
   A. Brainstem
   B. Spinal cord motor roots
   C. Cranial nerves
   D. Cerebral cortex

21. Occupational therapy services can be paid for under which part(s) of Medicare?
   A. Part A
   B. Part B
   C. Both A and B
   D. Only under supplemental insurance

22. Supervision is considered a professional responsibility and therefore a component of practice. Who is required to have supervision?
   A. All COTAs and entry-level OTRs
   B. Entry-level COTAs and OTRs
   C. Entry-level COTAs
   D. Entry-level OTRs

23. Examination of the efficiency of institutional use and the appropriateness of admissions, services, length of stay, and/or discharges is called:
   A. Continuous quality assurance
   B. Retrospective analysis
   C. Utilization review
   D. Fee monitoring

24. Which of the following is *not* present at birth?
   A. Moro reflex
   B. Symmetrical postures
   C. Babinski reflex
   D. Impassive facial expression

25. During an intake interview, a patient's ideas constantly shift from one subject to another. There is no apparent connection to his thoughts. This is called:
   A. Blocking
   B. Perseveration
   C. Flight of ideas
   D. Loose association

26. All the of the following are contraindications for aquatic therapy *except*:
   A. Open wound
   B. Decreased cardiovascular endurance
   C. Incontinence
   D. Severe cardiovascular disease

27. When making a forearm trough splint, the splint should be what length of the forearm?
   A. One fourth
   B. One third
   C. One half
   D. Two thirds

28. The *best* activity to assess motor synthesis is:
   A. Playing hopscotch
   B. Guessing an object's name without looking at it
   C. Constructing a three-dimensional box out of paper
   D. Copying a two-dimensional block design

29. All of the following activities are suited to increase spatial relationship awareness *except*:
    A. Making a tall tower of blocks
    B. Doing arithmetic problems
    C. Drawing hands on a clock
    D. Drawing a designated object from memory.

30. Your client has a dual diagnosis of hemiplegia and congestive heart failure. You anticipate fluctuating edema in the involved hemiplegic hand. What type of straps should you use on the client's splint?
    A. 1-inch wide webbing with a D ring
    B. 2-inch wide soft velcro
    C. 4-inch wide ace wrap
    D. Wide, soft, foam-like strap

31. The ability to derive meaning from an event or experience beyond the tangible aspects of the event itself is know as:
    A. Immediate recall
    B. Abstract thinking
    C. Concentration
    D. Attention

32. In order to increase a patient's compliance with splint usage after discharge, what is the *most* important factor?
    A. Listen to the patient's complaints and adjust splint
    B. Allow the patient to practice donning and doffing the splint
    C. Label the splint
    D. Contrast the colors of the splint and the straps

33. The *best* activity for persons with schizophrenia according to Lorna Jean King is:
    A. A routine exercise program
    B. Country line dancing
    C. Spontaneous movement to music
    D. Tap dancing

34. What neurological pathway in the brainstem is responsible for controlling consciousness and regulating the sleep-wake cycle?
    A. Basal ganglia
    B. Anterior corticospinal tract
    C. Lateral corticospinal tract
    D. Reticular formation

35. Which circuit within the basal ganglia has been implicated to be involved in obsessive-compulsive disorders?
    A. Motor circuit
    B. Oculomotor circuit
    C. Prefrontal association circuit
    D. Limbic circuit

36. An 84-year-old female nursing home resident is 5 years post CVA. Her left hand is in the fist-ed position and PROM is painful to her. Skin care is a concern. What is the *best* choice for intervention?
    A. None, nothing can be effectively done
    B. Daily soaks to relax the left hand and keep clean
    C. Resting hand splint
    D. Soft splint

 37. Post-traumatic stress disorder is *least* likely to be triggered by:
    A. Job loss
    B. Combat experience
    C. Sexual abuse
    D. Natural catastrophes

38. Intrinsics of the hand include all of the following *except*:
    A. Flexor pollicis longus
    B. Flexor digiti minimi
    C. Flexor pollicis brevis
    D. Abductor pollicis brevis

39. At what age can a child maintain head control when supported in sitting?
    A. 1 month
    B. 2 months
    C. 4 months
    D. 5 months

 40. A child of 2 to 3 years old grabs a chunky crayon with his fingers while his wrist is pronated is showing what type of grasp?
    A. Mature dynamic tripod
    B. Less mature static tripod
    C. Immature pronated grasp
    D. Power grasp

41. All of the following are spinal cord level reflexes *except*:
    A. Rooting, sucking
    B. Flexor withdrawal, placing
    C. Stepping, galant
    D. Asymmetric tonic neck reflex, symmetric tonic neck reflex

 42. The most common classification of cerebral palsy is:
    A. Spasticity
    B. Athetosis
    C. Flaccid/atonia
    D. Mixed

43. Developmental tasks of a person in later adulthood include all of the following *except*:
    A. Acceptance of one's self and life
    B. Acceptance of one's ethnic origin and identity
    C. Acceptance of one's mortality
    D. Acceptance of one's sexual identity

44. Tetraplegia is a term that indicates:
    A. The involvement of only the hands in plegia
    B. The involvement of only the lower extremities
    C. The involvement of only one side
    D. The involvement of four limbs

45. Post-polio syndrome can be associated with all of the following *except*:
    A. Weakness
    B. Fatigue
    C. Rapid onset of symptoms
    D. Chronic overuse resulting in limb pain

46. Pervasive development disorders include all of the following *except*:
    A. Autism
    B. Asperger's disorder
    C. Rett's disorder
    D. Childhood schizophrenia

47. A child in a full inclusion classroom requires staff and parent education to succeed. The role of the occupational therapist includes all of the following *except*:
    A. Educate the teacher on body mechanics so the teacher does not hurt her back when moving the child
    B. Educate the parents on techniques to maintain performance in the classroom
    C. Advise the parents on medical procedures that can enhance classroom performance
    D. Educate the teacher's aide to optimum classroom positioning and seating for the child

48. A 17-year-old young man with autism has been successful in all his occupational therapy treatments except shaving. His female classroom teacher reports some peers are teasing him about his "5 o'clock shadow." The teenager lives at home with his single mother and two younger sisters. The mother is frustrated because she has to nag the teen to get him to shave in the morning. As the school-based consulting OT, what is the *best* option for treatment:
    A. Have the teen wait to shave until he gets to school and then have his teacher supervise
    B. Allow the teen's beard to grow in and not shave at all
    C. Start a shaving group with all the young men in the teen's classroom
    D. Arrange a male teen volunteer to role model shaving with the young man

49. All of the following are foundations of spatiotemporal adaptation frame of reference *except*:
    A. Adaptation occurs with interaction of the individual and environment over time and space
    B. Spatiotemporal stress is both positive and negative
    C. Processing develops from reflex to motor planning
    D. Handling and positioning are used with inhibiting techniques

50. Sensory integration development continues throughout life but is generally complete by what age?
    A. 1 to 3 years of age
    B. 4 to 5 years of age
    C. 8 to 10 years of age
    D. 14 to 18 years of age

Section Three

1. What grasp pattern uses both thumb and fingers to hold an object against the palm?
   A. Lateral or key grasp
   B. Radial digit grasp
   C. Pad to pad grasp
   D. Cylindrical grasp

2. If you were asked to perform a neurological examination on a 40-year-old client with a CVA, what should you include in the evaluation?
   A. Coordination evaluation
   B. Apraxia evaluation
   C. Cognitive testing
   D. Perceptual evaluation

3. An entry-level COTA has the necessary knowledge to perform what type of evaluations?
   A. Perceptual
   B. Cognitive
   C. ADL
   D. Sensory motor

4. Medicare Part A pays for all *except*:
   A. Hospital inpatient stay
   B. Physician outpatient visits
   C. Skilled nursing facility
   D. Home and hospice care

5. Which assessment is *best* to evaluate motor skills in an adult?
   A. Adult Activity Inventory
   B. Purdue Pegboard
   C. Comprehensive Occupational Therapy Evaluation (COTE)
   D. Southern California Sensory Integration Tests (SCSIT)

6. ADA has had sweeping reforms in barrier-free designs. When planning the floor space of any department, what is the minimum width of a door frame?
   A. 28 inches
   B. 30 inches
   C. 32 inches
   D. 36 inches

7. Occupational therapy managers should develop departmental policies for all of the following reasons *except*:
   A. Policies clarify prohibited behaviors
   B. Policies negate the code of ethics
   C. Policies are guides to thinking and action
   D. Policies suggest courses of action

8. What activity is *best* to encourage cocontraction in children with low tone?
   A. Playing "Statue"
   B. Going through an obstacle course
   C. Pretending to ice skate around the room
   D. Finger painting

9. A life skills management group to increase functional skills would include all of the following *except*:
   A. Increasing conversations
   B. Food preparations
   C. Problem solving
   D. Money management

10. SOAP notes are sometimes used for documentation. In what section would the patient's comments during treatment go?
    A. Subjective (S)
    B. Objective (O)
    C. Assessment (A)
    D. Plan (P)

11. Where would you locate the acromion process?
    A. Humerus
    B. Clavicle
    C. Scapula
    D. Vertebrae

12. A deformity where the finger is positioned in extreme PIP flexion and DIP hyperextension is called:
    A. Ulnar deviation
    B. Boutonniere
    C. Swan neck
    D. Intrinsic plus

13. Your client is a 75-year-old female who has significant hyposensitivity in the left arm following a right CVA. The *most* important intervention for this client would be:
    A. Sensory re-education
    B. Safety and compensation instruction
    C. Motor and movement therapy of the left UE
    D. Self-care instructions with emphasis on the non-involved limb

14. What factor is *most* important in OT staff retention?
    A. High salaries
    B. Job satisfaction
    C. Continuing education opportunities
    D. Health insurance benefits

15. Research in occupational therapy is:
    A. Well-developed and complete
    B. Usually done with other disciplines
    C. In the early stages of growth and development
    D. Of little value because it is statistical in nature

16. Your client is a 6-year-old boy who is highly distractible. You have designed a very structured program aimed at providing a successful experience for the patient. Your environment should be:
    A. Bright colors with several choices of toys for fine motor skill development
    B. Distracting and competitive stimuli are low
    C. A simulated classroom
    D. No particular environmental factors need to be addressed due to the structured program

17. Capital expenses of an occupational therapy program might include:
    A. Land and buildings
    B. Supplies
    C. Equipment under $500.00
    D. OT staff salaries

18. The unconscious forgetting of an idea which is anxiety producing and unacceptable to the person in some way is known as:
    A. Dementia
    B. Repression
    C. Impaired judgment
    D. Regression

19. Which of the following statements is *not* true about psychotropic medication?
    A. Imipramine was the first tricyclic antidepressant to be discovered
    B. Thorazine signaled the beginning of modern psychopharmacology for antipsychotic medication
    C. Prozac is a relatively safe drug for treating schizophrenia
    D. Ritalin is effective in treating attention deficit disorder

20. Doorknobs should be placed at what height from the floor to allow for accessibility for people in wheelchairs?
    A. 28 inches
    B. 30 inches
    C. 32 inches
    D. 36 inches

21. The format for documentation is largely:
    A. Decided by management at the facility
    B. Agreed upon by majority rule within the OT department
    C. Outlined by regulation or law
    D. Developed by faculty from OT schools

22. Certification of a COTA is granted by:
    A. AOTA, AMA, and APA jointly
    B. COTA's own association
    C. State certification boards
    D. NBCOT

23. Your client is a 4-year-old girl with cerebral palsy and very low tone. When she is positioned in her customized wheelchair, her head is forward and she cannot maintain the vertical position. What is the *best* intervention?
    A. Recline the wheelchair so gravity will pull her head into neutral
    B. Give verbal commands to pull up her head
    C. Present an object in her visual field to elicit extension through eye tracking
    D. Use a soft cervical collar or molded neck collar to increase head control

24. The mother of a 5-year-old child with developmental delays tells you that she is unable to do his home care program because she is "too busy." You suspect that there might be other reasons. What should you do first?
    A. Emphasize the importance of the home program
    B. Discontinue the program and see the client in the clinic again
    C. Talk to the mother about problems she is facing
    D. Provide more information on how to make the home program easier

25. MMT is a valuable test of muscle power. It can also provide additional information on all of the following *except*:
    A. Resistance muscles can tolerate
    B. Muscle endurance
    C. ROM through which joints pass
    D. Gains or losses in strength

26. What disorder is characterized by the presence of one or more neurological symptoms such as paralysis, blindness, and/or paresis; has no known neurological or medical base; and psychological factors are associated with the initiation or exacerbation of symptoms?
    A. Hypochondriasis
    B. Korsakoff's syndrome
    C. Conversion disorder
    D. Dissociative identity disorder

27. Myopathies are a group of muscle diseases whose common principle symptom is generally proximal weakness. Which activity, if performed suboptimally, could indicate a myopathy?
    A. Eating a bowl of soup
    B. Climbing stairs
    C. Brushing teeth
    D. Donning pants

28. A person with a spinal cord injury who complains of dizziness and feels faint may be experiencing:
    A. Autonomic dysreflexia
    B. Pulmonary emboli
    C. Orthostatic hypotension
    D. Abdominal distention

29. Pressure ulcers are a concern in chronic rehabilitation. The *most* important consideration in the management of pressure ulcers is:
    A. Early detection
    B. Prevention
    C. Understanding potential signs
    D. Understanding friction force and support surfaces

30. Deep vein thrombi can result from all conditions *except*:
    A. Myocardial infarct
    B. Prolonged immobilization
    C. CVA/stroke
    D. Reflex sympathetic dystrophy

31. A person with a spinal cord injury who has active wrist extension and tenodesis function is at what level?
    A. C4
    B. C5
    C. C6
    D. C9

32. A client with a C5 spinal cord injury is ready to address self-feeding. What piece of equipment would the client benefit *most* from?
    A. Mobile arm support
    B. Universal cuff
    C. Electric wheelchair
    D. Scoop dish

33. In a pediatric population, what type of equipment is *most* effective for vestibular treatment?
    A. Suspended equipment
    B. ADL equipment
    C. Computer equipment
    D. Pen and paper tasks in a classroom

34. A blind or visually impaired person may have some sight. All of the following can assist the individual in his or her home environment *except*:
    A. A contrasting scatter rug by the doors
    B. A dark placemat or cup on a light surface
    C. Stair risers painted in a contrasting color
    D. White tape to mark a dark object

35. When a person has lost all vision, all of the following are helpful *except*:
    A. Textured surfaces to indicate the top and bottom of stairs
    B. Safety pins in different arrangements to mark clothes
    C. Textured doorknobs to mark exits
    D. Labels or signs in Braille

36. As part of managed health care, cross training is used. This involves:
    A. OTs cotreating the patient at the same time with a PT
    B. Many disciplines being able to meet the client's basic needs
    C. OTs continuing their education to avoid being laid off
    D. OTs being physical fit so they work at maximum efficiency

37. Critical paths are:
    A. Planned treatment schedules based on effective treatment approaches
    B. An environmental simulation that has different textures
    C. A warning that the patient may have an infectious disease
    D. Important documentation that is found in the front of the medical record

38. When should discharge plans begin?
    A. At admission
    B. Once the patient is out of the critical care unit
    C. When rehabilitation begins
    D. At least 1 week before the patient is ready for discharge

39. When a patient is frightened to transfer out of bed and into a wheelchair, the occupational therapist should do all of the following *except*:
    A. Use a firm touch and hurried motions to make the transfer as quick as possible
    B. Tell the patient what you intend to do and how you will do it
    C. Answer "I can't" with "Yes, you can, and I will help you"
    D. Instruct one step at a time

40. Basic body mechanics assist both the patient and the therapist. All of the following are good body mechanics *except*:
    A. When possible push, pull, or slide an object rather than pick it up
    B. Slight body twisting will provide more lift when picking up a heavy object
    C. Maintain your center of gravity (COG) close to the COG of the object you are holding
    D. Widen your base of support to stabilize your vertical gravity line

41. The best way to clean a wheelchair after it has been exposed to rain or snow is:
    A. Hose it down with clean water
    B. Let it air dry
    C. Use a light oil on the cross-brace center pin
    D. Wipe it dry with a cloth using a metal cleaner if needed

42. Severe swallowing disorders are associated with:
    A. High risk of aspiration
    B. Olfactory changes
    C. Nasal tumors
    D. Poor oral hygiene

43. A person with Alzheimer's disease who is unable to manage bathing but is still able to choose the proper clothing for the season might indicate a differential diagnosis of:
    A. Arthritis
    B. Schizophrenia
    C. Myocardial infarction
    D. Multiple sclerosis

44. Signs of extrapyramidal reactions include all of the following *except*:
    A. Lip puckering or smacking
    B. Inability to sustain tongue movement
    C. Frowning, blinking, smiling, or grimacing
    D. Arms rapidly moving without objective or slow athetoid movements

45. When teaching elderly clients about their medication routine, keep information short and to the point, be concrete about the time the medication should be taken, provide written directions at the end of the session, and:
    A. Use the words "drugs" or "pills" instead of the word "medicine"
    B. Ask the client to repeat information back to you
    C. Use technical words as well as common language
    D. Change all bottles to easy-open caps

46. Which of the following alternatives to restraints for the confused elderly is *not* effective?
    A. Structured, predictable routine
    B. Several activities to choose from
    C. Validate feelings, if resident is looking for mother, attend to the feelings behind it
    D. Place names and pictures on door

47. Which of the following alternatives to restraints for the wandering elderly is *not* effective?
    A. Opportunity for exercise
    B. Put bells on their shoes
    C. Safe, closed area outside or inside
    D. Identity bracelet

48. Mildred Ross's five-stage integrative group therapy includes orientation, movement activities, visual perceptual motor activities, cognitive activities, and:
   A. Closure activities to establish environmental trust
   B. Sensory integration activities
   C. Memory activities to stimulate abstract thinking
   D. Exercise to facilitate muscle tone

49. Activities that are alerting to the sensory integrative systems include all of the following *except*:
   A. Fast, loud music of variable intensity
   B. Swinging or sustained movements
   C. Light touch, whisking, brushing movements
   D. Increased muscle activities

50. Which assessment can be used in a geriatric setting providing information on a patient's independent activities of daily living and effective outcome measures as well?
   A. Kohlman Evaluation of Living Skills
   B. Barthel Index
   C. First STEp
   D. Peabody Developmental Motor Scale

Section Four

1. What reflex is developmentally appropriate until age 5 months, vital for newborns, and can be seen when the corner of the infant's mouth is stroked?
   A. Grasp reflex
   B. Galant reflex
   C. Primary righting action
   D. Rooting reflex

2. An individual member of AOTA in good standing is one who has done all of the following *except*:
   A. Paid membership fees
   B. Uphold the standards and ethics of the association
   C. Met the qualifications for membership
   D. Made a significant contribution to the profession

Use the following information to answer questions 3 and 4: During an occupational therapy task group, you observe your patient's cognitive abilities. George is able to complete a simple three-step craft project with visual cuing from the OTR at each step. While disregarding the written directions, George uses the sample project as a guide. His attention span is intact for 45 minutes.

3. According to Claudia Allen, at what level is your patient performing?
   A. Level 3, manual
   B. Level 4, goal directed
   C. Level 5, exploratory
   D. Level 6, planned

4. According to Allen, besides a simple craft project, what other activity would be *best* for George to work on cognitive functioning?
   A. Playing the game "Simon Says"
   B. Making a sandwich
   C. Budgeting for 1 day
   D. Making a model airplane that snaps together

5. When determining staff requirements for a new occupational therapy department, the *most* important factor to consider is:
   A. Patient load requirements
   B. Size of the space where OT will be housed
   C. The number of physical therapists there are
   D. Type of funding available

6. Membership to AOTA is open to:
   A. Occupational therapy students
   B. OTRs
   C. COTAs
   D. All the above

7. Occupational performance areas in Uniform Terminology include:
   A. Self-care
   B. Work
   C. Play/leisure
   D. All the above

8. You have just completed an ADL evaluation on a 65-year-old female. She had a right CVA in the nondominant hemisphere parietal lobe. During the evaluation you noticed the patient did dress the unaffected limb but did not dress the affected limb. This is an indication of:
   A. Apraxia motor
   B. Ideational apraxia
   C. Unilateral body neglect
   D. Astereognosis

9. Manual muscle testing should be performed on all patients *except*:
   A. C4 spinal cord injury
   B. Multiple sclerosis
   C. Spastic hemiplagia CVA
   D. Non-acute rheumatoid arthritis

   Use the following information to answer questions 10 and 11: Your client has third-degree burns on 18% of total body surface area (TBSA). He is very fearful of any movement of the involved areas.

10. How is TBSA calculated in burn patients over the age of 16?
    A. Skin burn depth is calculated
    B. Rule of nines, the body is divided into areas of 9%
    C. The physician decides with the help of the burn team
    D. The physician alone decides the level of involvement

11. How do you give the client encouragement to move or participate in therapy?
    A. Provide early ADL instruction
    B. Provide adaptive equipment
    C. Provide very structured regime of exercises
    D. Allow client to direct therapy, giving him control by doing AROM

12. The posterior rotator cuff muscles include:
    A. Supraspinatus, infraspinatus, and teres minor
    B. Subscapularis, infraspinatus, and teres major
    C. Sternocleidomastoid, infraspinatus, and teres major
    D. Subscapularis, infraspinatus, and triceps

13. A chronic and recurrent experience characterized by anxiety and often expressed through defense mechanisms which impairs one's life is called:
    A. Neuroses
    B. Psychoses
    C. Mental disorder
    D. Dysphoria

14. The registration exam for the OTR is administered by:
    A. AOTA
    B. NBCOT
    C. AOTF
    D. Each state's licensure board

15. Referral for occupational therapy services may come from:
    A. Physician
    B. Teacher
    C. Other therapists
    D. All the above

16. A person with C5 spinal cord injury would have all of the following muscle function *except*:
    A. Deltoids, shoulder flexion
    B. Biceps, elbow flexion
    C. Serratus anterior, scapular abduction
    D. Triceps, elbow extension

Use the following information to answer questions 17 through 19: Your 22-year-old male patient has Guillain-Barré syndrome. He has no speech, poor oral functioning, and all four limbs and trunk are severely involved. He has just been transferred from an acute care hospital to the rehabilitation hospital where you work.

17. Guillain-Barré syndrome is:
    A. A lower motor neuron disease
    B. A genetic disease
    C. A disease resulting from long-term abuse of alcohol
    D. A disease with total recovery

18. Symptoms of Guillain-Barré syndrome include all of the following *except*:
    A. Motor weakness and paralysis
    B. Sensory loss
    C. Compromised respiratory system
    D. Inflammation of the spinal cord

19. The *best* treatment for the first day in the rehabilitation hospital would be:
    A. Begin the evaluation but take frequent breaks
    B. Evaluate for and provide resting hand splints
    C. Set up a chin-operated communication device to call the nurse
    D. Educate the patient about occupational therapy

20. A newly admitted patient on the psychiatric unit develops a strong dislike for the OTR without provocation or incident. This is an example of:
    A. Consensual validation
    B. Therapist transparency
    C. Transference
    D. Counter transference

21. Which activity is *best* for a 10-year-old boy who needs facilitation of tactile input and kinesthetic awareness?
    A. Playing a board game
    B. Rubbing different textures on his arm
    C. Playing "Simon Says"
    D. Having the child stand beside a wall and roll one way then the other

22. The executive director of AOTA is:
    A. Employed by the national association
    B. Approves policies of AOTA
    C. Elected by the ethics committee of AOTA
    D. The chairperson of the representative assembly

23. An OTR receives a referral from a physician with a specific treatment recommendation. After evaluation of the patient, the OTR believes a different treatment would be more effective for the patient. The *best* course of action for the OTR is:
    A. Complete the different treatment, then call the physician
    B. Complete the original prescribed treatment, call the physician, and report that it is working
    C. Call the physician and suggest the OTR's treatment as an alternative to the prescription
    D. Combine the two treatments and hope one is effective

Use the following information to answer questions 24 and 25: One of the greatest dangers for a person with C4 spinal cord injury is autonomic dysreflexia. The occupational therapist must know how to recognize and manage this.

24. The symptoms of autonomic dysreflexia include all of the following *except*:
    A. Increased perspiration
    B. Flushing of the skin
    C. Dry, hot skin
    D. Severe headache

25. The *best* response if your client exhibits autonomic dysreflexia is:
    A. Keep the patient upright in the wheelchair and get immediate medical assistance
    B. Check the leg bag tubing for an obstruction, check blood pressure, and continue therapy if no problems are noted
    C. Recline the patient and get immediate medical assistance
    D. Ask someone to inform the nurse that the patient is complaining of a headache

26. All of the following are common pathological causes of feeding and swallowing disorders in the elderly *except*:
    A. Stroke
    B. Head trauma
    C. Liver or kidney disease
    D. Degenerative neurological disorders

27. The development of coma in a person with Alzheimer's disease can be the result of all of the following *except*:
    A. Myocardial infarction
    B. Overmedication
    C. Stroke
    D. Head trauma

28. Adverse drug reactions are common in the elderly. Which statement is *not true* about these reactions in older adults?
    A. Toxic reaction can occur even at low drug dosages
    B. Reactions can include drowsiness, depression, confusion, or dizziness
    C. Medications can cause involuntary movements or drug-related parkinsonism
    D. Over-the-counter drugs such as antacids, cold medicines, and laxatives are safe

29. Alternatives to restraining elderly residents who are unsteady on their feet include all of the following *except*:
    A. Address possible low vision problems
    B. Reading material or books on tapes
    C. Soft slippers and increased ambulation
    D. Meaningful activities to participate in

30. Activities that are calming to the sensory integrative systems include all of the following *except*:
    A. Defy gravity, up and down
    B. Swinging or sustained movements
    C. Heavy touch, massage
    D. Decreased motor activities

31. All of the following techniques are effective in the behavioral management of persons with brain injury *except*:
    A. Praise efforts of the client to regain control
    B. Give an alternative such as "I'll have to report this behavior to the team"
    C. Create a plan or agreement to accomplish tasks
    D. Ignore negative, attention-seeking behaviors and comments

32. At what age is the highest frequency of epilepsy seen?
    A. Birth to 10 years
    B. 11 to 39 years
    C. 40 to 69 years
    D. 70 years plus

33. Complications of spasticity include all of the following *except*:
    A. Hypotonic muscles around joints leads to poor support
    B. Poor skin hygiene
    C. Contractures
    D. Decubiti

34. The following clinical signs are noted in your patient: ataxic gait, hypotonia, dysmetria, and dysdiadochokinesia. From these clinical signs, which part of the brain has sustained damage?
    A. Parietal lobe
    B. Premotor cortex
    C. Cerebellum
    D. Basal ganglia

35. An example of an eclectic frame of reference is:
    A. Behavior modification
    B. Object relations
    C. Cognitive behavioral
    D. Task-oriented treatment

36. What would be the *best* treatment options for a child with sensory integration, particularly vestibular problems?
    A. Reading a book in a big, overstuffed chair in the library
    B. Playing on the fixed monkey bars in the schoolyard
    C. Playing on the swing set in the schoolyard
    D. Being wrapped up tight in a blanket in a comfortably warm room

37. All of the following statements are true concerning phantom sensation following limb loss in adults *except*:
    A. Almost all adults experience phantom sensations following limb loss
    B. 60% of all patients experience phantom pain
    C. Phantom pain is considered a disturbance in body image
    D. The existence of neurological scheme ends with the actual physical loss of the limb

38. A patient with left-sided hemiplegia is asked to draw a clock. All of the following are being evaluated *except*:
    A. Visual perception
    B. Visual sequencing
    C. Visual constructive ability
    D. Ability to tell time

39. Which assessment is designed to identify developmental delays of preacademic skills in children?
    A. Movement Assessment of Infants Screening Test
    B. Erhardt Developmental Prehension Assessment
    C. Miller Assessment for Preschoolers
    D. Peabody Developmental Motor Scales

40. What would be the *best* cognitive behavioral activity to use in occupational therapy?
    A. One that teaches ADL skills with emphasis on education and successful completion
    B. One that increases sensory input and facilitates an adaptive response
    C. One that identifies activities for fulfilling occupational roles
    D. One that emphasizes art and drawing with the meaning of symbols

41. Which of the following statements is *true* about spasticity?
    A. May aid in the prevention of osteoporosis
    B. May aid in the prevention of muscle atrophy
    C. Prevention of deep vein thrombosis
    D. All the above

42. The assessment of cognition includes attention, orientation, memory, mental status, and:
    A. Executive function
    B. Motor apraxia
    C. Perceptual function
    D. Visual motor function

43. Gradation of an activity means:
    A. Assigning a grade to the patient's completed task
    B. Adjusting the pace and modifying the demand to meet the patient's maximum capabilities
    C. Assigning minimal to maximum assistance to the task depending on the amount of assistance
       the patient needs from the therapist
    D. Encouraging the patient to try one more time to complete an uncompleted task

44. All of the following demonstrate good listening skills *except*:
    A. Lean slightly backwards
    B. Make eye contact
    C. Body appears open
    D. Face client squarely

Use the following information to answer questions 45 through 48: You are an occupational therapist working in a specialized facility for people with head traumas. Your facility treats clients from subacute to community reentry and outpatient. The facility uses Rancho Los Amigos (RLA) levels to assign clients to different programs. You have clients in all the different programs.

45. When working with patients with head injuries, what level does sensory stimulation treatment seem most appropriate?
    A. Level I
    B. Level III
    C. Level V
    D. Level VII

46. When would the same sensory stimulation treatment be the *most in*appropriate?
    A. Level I
    B. Level II
    C. Level III
    D. Level IV

47. At what level is repetition and practice of tasks *most* appropriate?
    A. Level IV
    B. Level V
    C. Level VI
    D. Level VII

48. Level VIII is purposeful and appropriate interaction with the environment. All of the following would be effective treatment for a client at level VIII *except*:
    A. Cognitive rehabilitation
    B. Vocational rehabilitation
    C. Work hardening programs
    D. Community mobility training

49. The *best* response to a person who is clearly psychotic, telling you how the FBI and CIA are chasing him, is:
    A. "I have to go now"
    B. "That's very interesting, tell me more about that"
    C. "Now think about this, you know it can't be true, it's part of your disease"
    D. "That sounds crazy to me, I can't talk to you when you say these things"

50. Which activity is *most* appropriate for a person hearing threatening voices?
    A. A 1,000-piece puzzle
    B. A tie-dyed t-shirt
    C. Leather wallet with written directions
    D. Learning a simple word processing computer program

Section Five

1. Low back pain is a common problem for most of the adult population. The aging process results in loss of water in the disc and the joint space narrows. What role does occupational therapy play in reducing the risk of back injury?
    A. Teaching strengthening programs
    B. Redesigning work stations
    C. Observation of client body mechanics
    D. Prevention and retraining education

2. Your client experienced a myocardial infarction 3 days ago and is feeling anxious. He is medically stable and his doctor has explained what has happened, but the client remains anxious. What is the *best* approach for rehabilitation of this client?
    A. Educate the family to client's decrease in activity tolerance
    B. Teach client energy conservation and work simplification
    C. Begin graded resistive exercise program
    D. Stress reduction and long-term relaxation techniques

3. The BTE is an electromagnetic device that has 20 interchangeable tools and utilizes a computer to calibrate and calculate data in a qualitative way. For what type of program is this piece of equipment ideal?
   A. Cardiac rehabilitation
   B. CVA motor learning program
   C. Work rehabilitation
   D. Sensory integration programs

4. Play is often seen as child's work. Children who do not play are ill-prepared for adulthood. In the hospital the OTR should foster play by doing all of the following *except*:
   A. Structure the activities to prevent spontaneous play
   B. Role model the excitement of exploration
   C. Alternate solitary activity with social activity
   D. Have activities to develop problem solving and decision making

5. An OTR is asked to give a presentation to a local advocacy group for adults with mental health problems. The *most* effective presentation would be:
   A. Reviewing assessments such as BaFPE, ACL, KELS
   B. Discussing problems that adults with mental health diagnoses might have and how occupational therapy addresses those problems
   C. A demonstration of new computer programs to refer patients to community placements
   D. Teaching basic counseling techniques so the audience can use them with their consumers

6. What governmental program provides medical coverage for people age 65 and over?
   A. Medicaid
   B. Medicare
   C. SSI/SSD
   D. Welfare and section 8

7. The purpose of documentation includes all of the following *except*:
   A. Data for research, education, reimbursement, treatment
   B. Serial and legal record of therapeutic intervention
   C. Facilitate communication among health care professionals
   D. Cover the therapist in case there is an ethical problem

Use the following information to answer questions 8 and 9: A 25-year-old female psychiatric patient puts on dark sunglasses every time she passes you in the hallway. During your initial OT assessment, you ask her about this behavior. She tells you that the glasses prevent you from putting horrible thoughts in her head.

8. This behavior is an example of:
   A. Thought insertion
   B. Delusions of reference
   C. Hypervigilance
   D. Magical thinking

9. The *most* appropriate response for the OTR would be:
   A. "That's true"
   B. "Why would you think that?"
   C. "It is inappropriate to wear sunglasses indoors"
   D. "You must be feeling uneasy with me in this interview"

10. A needs assessment can provide information about the need for a new occupational therapy program. All of the following are good sources of information *except*:
    A. Focus group of patients
    B. Survey to physicians
    C. Demographic information
    D. Etiology information

11. RSD is a debilitating, progressive disease. Your client is in the first stage of RSD with classic signs of hand edema, fear of ROM, and shoulder and hand pain. What is your first priority in treatment?
    A. Reduction of edema
    B. AROM with emphasis on self ROM
    C. Aggressive PROM to prevent stage II progression
    D. Establish rapport with patient while talking about ADLs

12. Occupational therapists can assess peripheral nerve function in their clients with many quick screening tests available to clinicians. The simple test for radial nerve function would be:
    A. Thumb and little finger opposition
    B. Wrist extension
    C. Gross grasp assessment with dynamometer
    D. Pinch thumb and index finger

13. Personality factors such as rigidity, hostility, manipulation, passive-aggressive, and dependent behaviors are associated with:
    A. Arthritis
    B. Multiple sclerosis
    C. Chronic pain syndrome
    D. All patients coping with chronic pain or chronic disabilities

14. Swan neck deformity can result from a rupture of the lateral slips of the extensor digitorum communis (EDC) tendon. What finger position would result?
    A. MCP subluxation
    B. DIP hyperextension and PIP flexion
    C. MCP ulnarly deviated
    D. PIP hyperextension and DIP flexion

Use the following information to answer questions 15 through 18: John is a 24-year-old single male recently admitted to the inpatient psychiatric unit. He lives at home with his parents and depends on them for financial support because he spends all his money. He presents as agitated, with sporadic concentration and racing thoughts. He believes that he is a famous rock star and is shocked that you do not recognize him. He says he cannot wait to start a project in OT.

15. John's symptoms *most* closely resemble which disorder?
    A. Obsessive-compulsive disorder
    B. Generalized anxiety disorder
    C. Bipolar disorder
    D. Attention deficit hyperactivity disorder

16. John's belief that he is a rock star is an example of:
    A. A hallucination
    B. A delusion, grandiose type
    C. Paranoid ideation
    D. Malingering

17. Which of the following would be the *most* appropriate goal for this patient?
    A. Increase decision making
    B. Improve level of independence in ADLs
    C. Improve socialization
    D. Increase self-control

18. Which of the following activities would be the *most* appropriate to begin treatment?
    A. A tile box
    B. A 2,000-piece puzzle
    C. Wood carving
    D. Budgeting

19. Your client has extensive burns involving the anterior aspect of the UE including the neck. Considering the position of comfort, what splint(s) would be indicated?
    A. Neck conformer
    B. Neck conformer, axillary
    C. Neck conformer, axillary, three-point elbow extension
    D. Neck conformer, axillary, three-point elbow extension, hand cock-up

20. The cause of incomplete flexion ROM of the MCP, PIP, and DIP while the wrist is in flexion is:
    A. Active insufficiency
    B. Passive insufficiency
    C. Decreased muscle strength
    D. Unknown

21. What activity is *best* to encourage the integration of primitive postural reflexes in a child?
    A. Have child lie prone on a scooter board and spin
    B. Have child walk on a balance beam
    C. Have child pretend to be a dog, crawl around, roll over, and bark
    D. Have child play a game of marbles

22. The NBCOT registration exam can be taken:
    A. After all classwork is finished
    B. After all fieldwork is finished
    C. After all classwork and fieldwork are finished
    D. After filing for licensure

23. What do the initials MORE stand for in OBRA regulations?
    A. Measurable, observable, reportable, exit behavior
    B. Measurable, observable, reportable, emotional
    C. Measurable, observable, realistic, explicit
    D. Measurable, observable, realistic, effective

24. When developing a new program for an already standing OT department, where would be the first place to start?
    A. Philosophy and mission statement
    B. Goals and objectives
    C. Patient services
    D. Documentation necessary

25. Scoliosis is defined as a:
    A. Narrowing of the lumbar spinal canal
    B. Gradual slipping of one vertebra on another
    C. Lateral curvature of the spine
    D. Chronic inflammation of the joints of the axial skeleton

26. Which sensory integration assessment requires additional training and certification to administer?
    A. Sensory Rating Scale
    B. Sensory Integration and Praxis Test
    C. Sensory Assessment
    D. Knickerbocker Sensorimotor History Questionnaire

27. People with Parkinson's disease often are given medication that is dopamine based which improves movement, however, as dopamine increases what side effect also increases?
    A. Cog wheel movements
    B. Unsteady gait
    C. Psychotic features
    D. Confusion

28. People usually do not realize this but most human beings hold their breath when they bend over to pick up something, tie their shoe, or garden. Which population is this particularly dangerous to?
    A. Cardiac patients
    B. Multiple sclerosis
    C. Orthopedic conditions
    D. Arthritis patients

29. The approximate percent of individuals with epilepsy who can be successfully treated with antiepileptic medications is:
    A. 10%
    B. 50%
    C. 80%
    D. 100%

30. According to the American Spinal Injury Association, the term "central cord syndrome" indicates:
    A. Greater weakness in the upper extremity than the lower
    B. Greater ipsilateral proprioceptive/motor loss and contralateral loss of temperature/pin sensitivity
    C. Loss of motor function but proprioception is intact
    D. Injury to the lumbosacral nerve roots with lower extremity involvement

31. The use of aquatic therapy is on the rise. The basic principle of this modality is buoyancy. If your 25-year-old patient with head trauma weighs 250 lbs on land, what is his approximate weight in the water?
    A. 225 lbs
    B. 175 lbs
    C. 125 lbs
    D. 75 lbs

32. You receive a referral from a classroom teacher to test a 7-year-old girl who the teacher suspects possible perceptual problems are leading to difficulty in reading. The child has spastic cerebral palsy but has kept up with her peers until now. What is the best test to use?
    A. Developmental Test of Visual Perception (DTVP-2)
    B. Test of Visual Motor Skills (TVMS)
    C. Test of Visual Perceptual Skills (TVPS)
    D. Motor-Free Visual Perception Test (MVPT)

33. AOTPAC is the political action committee that represents the profession of occupational therapy. AOTPAC suggests all occupational therapists must take an active role in national legislation that affects occupational therapy. When writing a letter to your Congressperson or your Senator:
    A. Explain how the issue will impact you and your community
    B. Avoid form letters
    C. Be constructive in your proposals, offering professional advice
    D. All of the above

34. You are about to treat a patient bedside but "Methicillin Resistant Staphylococcus Aureus" (MRSA) is noted in his chart. What does this mean?
    A. The patient is an IV abusing or recreational drug user
    B. The patient is ventilator dependent and requires oxygen monitoring
    C. The patient has an infection that cannot be treated with traditional antibiotics
    D. The patient is HIV positive and requires the use of universal precautions

35. Which assessment is *least* appropriate for evaluating independent living skills?
    A. Assessment of Motor and Process Skills (AMPS)
    B. Bay Area Functional Performance Evaluation (BaFPE)
    C. Older Americans Resources and Services Instrument (OARS)
    D. Fugl-Meyer Scale (FM)

36. What is the first thing a therapist should do when washing his or her hands?
    A. Turn on the water and adjust the temperature
    B. Apply soap to hands
    C. Remove rings and put them on the sink's edge
    D. Pull out a length of paper towel

37. If assessment on the Baltimore Therapeutic Equipment (BTE) simulator suggests that the maximum a female worker's compensation client can lift at this time is 7 lbs, which item in her home will she be unable to lift?
    A. A jumbo box of cereal
    B. A gallon of milk
    C. A blow dryer
    D. A portable telephone

38. Understanding an individual's weight bearing precautions is essential to addressing mobility with a client. Which level allows a small amount of weight to be applied by the affected leg?
    A. Toe touch weight bearing (TTWB)
    B. Partial weight bearing (PWB)
    C. Weight bearing as tolerated (WBAT)
    D. Full weight bearing (FWB)

39. Rotter introduced a concept which describes one's belief in personal responsibility for an outcome of an action. When a person believes that he or she is personally responsible for life events rather than life events being controlled by outside influences, this is called:
    A. Competence
    B. Locus of control
    C. Internal locus of control
    D. External locus of control

40. The term that defines the level of proficiency in a specific activity or task is known as:
    A. Skill
    B. Ability
    C. Autonomy
    D. Order

41. Which of the following outcomes or goals is applicable to Claudia Allen's cognitive disabilities frame of reference?
    A. To achieve competence in social roles
    B. To achieve mastery of developmental milestones
    C. To increase organization, function, and adaptation in occupational performance
    D. To improve thinking and performance in various activities

Use the following information to answer questions 42 through 44: Your client is a 64-year-old woman with rheumatoid joint disease. She is currently being seen three times a week in an outpatient program. The client exhibits multiple joint involvement in the wrist and hands. Currently in the clinic, the client is using paraffin, exercises, and experimenting with adaptive equipment. In addition, the client is participating in her home program. Presently, the client is on NSAIDs and a DMARD (a disease-modifying antirheumatic drug).

42. NSAIDs are:
    A. Nonsteroid anti-inflammatory drug
    B. Expensive medication
    C. New steroid anti-inflammatory drug
    D. Another disease-modifying drug

43. The client is reporting good results from her medication with decreased pain and stiffness, however, the client is reporting a skin rash on her arms and legs. The *best* course of action is to:
    A. Question the client's response to the paraffin and discontinue the use
    B. Question if the client is experiencing a side effect of the disease-modifying drug
    C. Question the client about past allergic reactions to aspirin or NSAIDs
    D. Consult with a family member regarding possible exposure to home contaminates

44. What is the *first* priority in choosing a piece of adaptive equipment for this particular client?
    A. A longhandled reacher so she does not have to reach so far
    B. A longhandled bath sponge to make showering easier
    C. A bar stool in the kitchen so she can rest during homemaking chores
    D. A piece of equipment that the client wants to use

45. Parkinson's disease is a movement disorder characterized by all of the following symptoms *except*:
    A. Postural instability
    B. Bradykinesia
    C. Rigidity
    D. Intentional tremor

46. What is the lowest level of OTR that can provide supervision of OT aides, technicians, care extenders, all levels of COTAs, volunteers, and Level I fieldwork students?
    A. Entry-level OTRs with less than 1 year experience
    B. Intermediate level OTRs
    C. Advance level OTRs with 5 or more years' experience
    D. Any physical therapist

47. An entry-level COTA with less than 1 year of experience must have close supervision by an OTR or intermediate/advanced COTA. How is close supervision defined?
    A. Constant, direct supervision of all treatment sessions
    B. Daily, direct contact at the work site
    C. Direct contact at least every 2 weeks with telephone contact more often
    D. Direct contact once a month with telephone contact as needed

48. An OTR works in a school system with children who have deficits in sensory integration. The OTR is utilizing A. J. Ayers' frame of reference to improve sensory integrative function and performance. How will this goal be *best* achieved?
    A. By controlling sensory input to elicit an adaptive response
    B. Through movement patterns requiring new responses
    C. Through direct involvement in activities that will develop work skills later in life
    D. Through stimulating task and interpersonal skill development

49. According to the World Health Organization International Classification, what is the correct definition of disability?
    A. Abnormality or loss pertaining to either psychological or physical origin
    B. Restriction to perform an activity within a normal range of functioning
    C. A disadvantage which limits or prevents fulfillment of normal role performance
    D. Disruption in the roles of daily living

50. The AOTA position paper on the use of physical agent modalities (PAMs) would allow the use of paraffin in all of the following cases *except*:
    A. As a warm-up for exercise for a client with a hand trauma
    B. Combined with other PAMs as a pain reliever
    C. Before doing keyboarding with a client with arthritis
    D. While trying to increase ROM in an elbow with chronic pain

Section Six

1. What is the *best* approach to prevent hypertrophic scarring of a patient with burns?
    A. The physical and occupational therapists would both range the patient daily
    B. The occupational therapist would splint the involved areas and measure the patient for pressure garments to be worn 23 hours per day
    C. Nursing would position the patient when not in therapy to prevent deformity
    D. The family would be involved to encourage the patient to comply with the rehabilitation program

2. Motor apraxia would be the *most* likely deficit when the patient:
    A. Attempts to grasp a washcloth and is unable to plan and sequence the hand movements
    B. Does not discern the foreground from the background and cannot find the soap or washcloth
    C. Becomes frustrated when having trouble with the task
    D. Did not comprehend the verbal instructions

3. Flaccidity or hypotonicity following a cerebral or spinal insult will include all of the following *except*:
    A. Decreased muscle tone
    B. Weak cocontractions
    C. Hyperactive tendon reflexes
    D. Decreased ability to resist gravity

4. A client with traumatic brain injury is in an outpatient program with the long-term goal of returning to work as an auto mechanic installing mufflers. Motorically the client is exhibiting good overall strength and coordination. In groups, he is unable to work with others or to control inappropriate behaviors. His occupational therapy program should include:
    A. Work program that includes muffler installations
    B. Pre work hardening with emphasis on social skills for work readiness
    C. Continued work on impulse control in an inpatient hospital setting
    D. Patient is appropriate for any work program at this time

5. Group members develop standards of participation for members and expectations for leaders. What is this called?
   A. Group norms
   B. Group roles
   C. Subgrouping
   D. Task roles

6. Vestibular stimulation when used to treat a child with autism is *least* effective for improving which of the following?
   A. Communication
   B. Hyporesponsiveness
   C. Self-care
   D. Muscle tone

7. When evaluating your client's ROM, you first ask her to move the part through available AROM. What do you learn about the client through your observation?
   A. The end feel of the joint
   B. That muscle strength is good because she achieved full AROM
   C. That muscle strength is fair or above if she achieved full AROM
   D. The joint passive or accessory play

8. The relationship between the vestibular system and the cerebellum has resulted in therapy concepts that suggest slow rocking and inversion will result in:
   A. Reduced hypotonicity
   B. Increased hypertonicity
   C. Reduced hypertonicity
   D. Increased hypotonicity

9. Diarthrodial or synovial joints include all of the following *except*:
   A. Ball and socket
   B. Hinge
   C. Saddle
   D. Suture

10. A contraction that occurs with muscle lengthening is known as:
    A. Concentric
    B. Isometric
    C. Eccentric
    D. Isotonic

11. Which of the following does *not* describe an example of social reinforcement?
    A. Making eye contact
    B. Smiling
    C. Therapeutic self-disclosure
    D. Nodding

nt is coming to OT to inhibit tonic neck reflex and to increase vestibular
he child to roll in a carpeted barrel or inner tube with handles. What pre-
ant?

watching will think the activity is unsafe

...at children may think of the barrel as a weapon

C. Be aware of too much pressure on the child's hips and legs

D. Be aware of too much vestibular input and the emotional responses

13. Which statement defines "process" in groups?
    A. Therapeutic dynamics
    B. Understanding the nature of interpersonal relationships
    C. Explicit words spoken by the members
    D. Therapeutic intervention

14. What do the initials POMR stand for?
    A. Problem-oriented medical record
    B. Performance-oriented medical record
    C. Problem-observation medical record
    D. Patient-oriented medical record

15. A client who has severe rheumatoid arthritis, but is currently in remission, wants to engage in
    a strengthening program. What type of exercises would be most beneficial?
    A. Concentric
    B. Eccentric
    C. Isotonic
    D. Isometric

16. During supination, what is moving?
    A. Ulna
    B. Radius
    C. Both ulna and radius
    D. Only the distal ulna

17. DRGs often influence hospital stay. What do the initials stand for?
    A. Diagnosis rate guide
    B. Determined and related groups
    C. Doctor's rate guide
    D. Diagnosis related groups

18. Your client has an above elbow amputation. He is fearful and hesitant to don his prosthetic
    device. What approach would be *most* helpful to the client?
    A. Wait until the client is ready to learn
    B. Work on a strengthening program instead
    C. Repetitive donning and removal of the prosthesis
    D. Work on stump care

19. A patient with recent hip replacement must avoid all of the following *except*:
    A. Bending while sitting
    B. Walking outside
    C. Crossed legs
    D. Crossed ankles

20. According to Anne Mosey, there are five types of nonfamilial groups simulating normal development. These groups can be organized in specific sequence to resemble the development of group interaction skills. Which of the following is *not* the correct name?
    A. Parallel
    B. Cooperative
    C. Project
    D. Egocentric

21. Occupational therapists can refer patients to:
    A. Physical therapists only in their facility
    B. Any health care professional as appropriate
    C. Only another OTR
    D. Only back to the doctor the patient originally had

22. Hypertension is easily detected by:
    A. Shortness of breath
    B. Headache
    C. Monitoring blood pressure with a sphygmomanometer
    D. Dizziness

23. Poor splint construction can lead to impaired function. The *most* important factor in custom splint construction is:
    A. Cosmetics—If it looks bad the client will have poor compliance
    B. During the molding, pay special attention to maintaining the arches
    C. Price—If it is too expensive the client will have poor compliance
    D. The materials used as straps

24. According to the model of human occupation frame of reference, what subsystem includes values and interests as components?
    A. Volitional
    B. Habituation
    C. Performance
    D. Environment

25. The *most* appropriate and inclusive evaluation to use with a patient suspected to have delirium would be:
    A. Allen's Cognitive Level (ACL)
    B. Bay Area Functional Performance Evaluation (BaFPE)
    C. Kohlman Evaluation of Living Skills (KELS)
    D. Mini Mental Status

cal agent modalities (PAMs) states that OT personnel are
...ve to or in preparation of purposeful activity *except*:

□

83

...ble to do them
...for the service

...rkinson's disease is associated with one main medica-

... (Levodopa)
C. NSAIDs
D. Heparin

28. A 30-year-old female waitress worked very long hours. One evening she fell asleep resting on her right forearm. She awoke 5 hours later with signs of radial nerve injury including wrist drop. Which splint is the *best* option for treatment?
   A. Resting hand splint
   B. Dynamic extension splint
   C. Radial gutter splint
   D. Ulnar gutter splint

29. What is the area in front of the eyes in which an object can be seen without moving the eyes?
   A. Cornea
   B. Retina
   C. Visual acuity
   D. Visual field

30. An OTR has just received a referral from a physician within an acute care hospital. What is the *first* step the OTR should take in problem solving the treatment process?
   A. Determine the patient's needs
   B. Write the treatment plan
   C. Assess the patient's strengths and weaknesses
   D. Plan possible intervention strategies

31. In a feeding program, puréed foods may be difficult for some clients to swallow for all of the following reasons *except*:
   A. Spicy or intense taste
   B. Unappealing appearance
   C. Lack of temperature and texture
   D. Minimal pressure requirements to chew

32. When a person with Alzheimer's cannot handle his finances but is still able to handle a demanding work schedule, what differential diagnosis might be present?
   A. Other forms of dementia in addition to Alzheimer's
   B. Pseudo dementia due to depression
   C. CVA
   D. Anoxia from COPD

33. What over-the-counter medications are contraindicated for a person in cardiac rehabilitation?
   A. Vitamins
   B. Aspirin
   C. Tylenol brand pain relievers
   D. Alka Seltzer brand stomach and cold remedies

34. What developmental stage is marked by the drive for independence, building social relation-ships, defining occupational/social roles, development of intellectual skills, and values/ethics?
   A. Childhood
   B. Adolescence
   C. Young adulthood
   D. Middle adulthood

35. A patient in occupational therapy continues to deny the seriousness of his diabetes. This typi-cal use of denial by physically ill people may be called what type of coping strategy?
   A. Cognitive strategy
   B. Behavioral strategy
   C. Avoidant strategy
   D. Problem-focused coping

36. Higher level cognitive skills, localized in the frontal lobes, are also called executive functions. All of the following are executive skills *except*:
   A. Initiation of action
   B. Ability to recognize and correct one's behavior
   C. Evaluation of one's ability with an expected performance standard
   D. Verbal discussion of desired behavior

Use the following information to answer questions 37 through 39: Your patient is a 70-year-old woman with a long history of congestive heart failure caused by myocarditis. She has been suc-cessfully treated with digitalis glycosides for several years. Some swelling is noted in her ankles and feet. Her endurance is slightly limited. She recently developed some weakness and incoordi-nation in her right side.

37. Her diagnosis is likely:
   A. Myocardial infarct
   B. Pulmonary edema
   C. CVA
   D. Additional congestive heart failure

38. The client was not hospitalized but will receive therapy at home. The OT priority would be?
   A. Increase strength and ROM in right UE
   B. Increase ADL status, especially dressing
   C. Client-centered therapy
   D. Home management

39. After 2 weeks of home therapy, you notice the client is confused and lethargic although there are no changes in her current motoric status. The *best* therapeutic response is:
   A. Continue to monitor the client's motoric status
   B. Consult with the family
   C. Consult with your OT supervisor
   D. Consult with the client's physician

40. Which law specifically prohibits discrimination solely based on an individual's disability in any program receiving federal monies?
   A. Rehabilitation Act of 1973, section 504
   B. Education of the Handicapped Act
   C. Americans with Disabilities Act
   D. PL 94-103

41. Vertical righting reactions in children:
   A. Activate muscles to move the midline of the body into alignment with the center of gravity
   B. Activate muscles to lift the head to either side
   C. Are present at birth
   D. All of the above

42. When a child is supported in the supine position and his head is gently dropped, what reflex elicits abduction and extension of arms followed by arms coming together in an arc?
   A. Flexor withdrawal
   B. Crossed extension
   C. Moro
   D. Bauer's

43. Enabling a person to interact with the environment effectively and develop an accurate map of self requires all of the following systems *except*:
   A. Olfactory
   B. Somatosensory
   C. Proprioceptive
   D. Vestibular

44. All of the following are true of psychoanalytic theory and its relationship to Fidler's task group *except*:
   A. Intrapsychic conflicts are explored
   B. Emphasis is placed on the success of the end product
   C. Unmasking the unconscious is encouraged through the activity process
   D. Freud is the father of psychoanalysis

45. For a college or university to offer an entry-level degree in occupational therapy, the program must meet:
   A. Essentials and guidelines for an accredited educational program for the occupational therapist
   B. Core values and attitudes of occupational therapy practice
   C. Standards of practice for occupational therapy
   D. Occupational therapy code of ethics

46. A patient who believes he cannot meet the therapist's expectations in skill performance and who fears criticism is most likely to refuse to attend which type of occupational therapy group?
    A. Weekend planning group (leisure)
    B. Community trip to the mall (socialization)
    C. Current events group (psychoeducational)
    D. Arts and crafts (task)

47. AOTA defines occupational therapy practitioners as:
    A. An OTR
    B. An OTR and COTA
    C. An OTR, COTA, or OT aide
    D. Any person who practices occupational therapy

48. The *Occupational Therapy Roles* paper is an official document of the AOTA. What roles are defined in this document?
    A. OTR and COTA practitioners
    B. Clinical and education fieldwork educators
    C. Supervisor, administrator, consultant, and entrepreneur
    D. All of the above

49. An occupational therapy group that has as its goal to increase the patient's planning and participation in self-care, work, and leisure is called:
    A. Coping skills
    B. Self-expression
    C. Time management
    D. Value clarification

50. A client diagnosed with narcissistic personality disorder has made a personal, sexual comment about you during occupational therapy group. What counseling strategy should you use?
    A. Self-disclosure to let the client know how offended you are by the comment
    B. Empathy to be considerate and convey understanding of the client's perspective
    C. Termination to expect the client to automatically leave your group
    D. Immediacy to discuss the therapeutic relationship and the impact on the both of you

Section Seven

1. Which of the following is *not* true about delirium and dementia?
    A. Both include cognitive impairment
    B. Incoherent speech may result
    C. Clouding of consciousness occurs
    D. Insight may be impaired

2. Your patient is about to be discharged home within a few days. He has described a long history of dependency on alcohol and cocaine for pleasure. It is apparent to you that his family and friends also have similar patterns of abuse. What would be the *best* treatment goal considering this environment?
    A. Increase problem solving
    B. Leisure planning
    C. Increase grooming/hygiene
    D. Identify values

s the end of the infancy stage of development?

rs
l

4. The *most* important role of AOTF is:
   A. Developing scholarships for OT students
   B. Facilitating a foundation and developing research in occupational therapy
   C. Fundraising for their own budget
   D. Housing the occupational therapy library

5. ROM is measured by placing the goniometer over the axis of the movement of the joint. When measuring glenohumeral shoulder flexion, the stationary arm of the goniometer would be positioned where?
   A. Parallel to the humerus
   B. Medial aspect of the ulna
   C. Longitudinal axis of the radius
   D. Parallel to the lateral midline of the trunk

6. The *most* important goal in teaching ADLs to a patient with LE, above knee amputation is:
   A. Use of adaptive equipment
   B. How to supervise others who help with home management
   C. Energy conservation and work simplification
   D. Cognitive retraining

7. A rotator cuff injury would result in clinical features that include:
   A. No restrictions in AROM of the shoulder
   B. Painful arch 50° to 100° and restricted AROM in shoulder abduction and flexion
   C. Total restriction in AROM of the shoulder
   D. Only full PROM would indicate restrictions

Use the following information to answer questions 8 and 9: During a coping skills activity in an inpatient psychiatric unit, your patient suddenly starts sweating, complains of his heart pounding, feels dizzy, and fears he is losing control. He suddenly runs out of the group.

8. These symptoms *most* likely describe:
   A. Generalized anxiety
   B. A heart attack
   C. Panic attack
   D. Stress

9. The OTR's *best* initial response would be:
   A. Encourage patient to return
   B. Notify other team members
   C. Remain with the group members
   D. Check on patient directly

10. When testing scapula elevation, which two muscles would be palpated?
    A. The rhomboids
    B. Sternocleidomastoid and upper trapezius
    C. Upper trapezius and levator scapula
    D. Pectoralis major and minor

11. The certification exam for the COTA is:
    A. The same as the OTR exam but COTAs have more time
    B. Different from the OTR exam
    C. The same as the OTR exam but easier to pass
    D. The same as the OTR but given on different days

12. Ataxia results in a lack of postural stability. If a client can ambulate but has ataxia and fatigue, what would you recommend while preparing meals in the kitchen?
    A. A home program of postural stability exercises
    B. Energy conservation and work simplification education
    C. The client should use a wheelchair in the kitchen
    D. A home health aide should take care of meal preparation

13. Spinal reflexes are considered to be more primitive and are noted for their quick action and extinction. They include all of the following *except*:
    A. Flexor withdrawal
    B. Extensor thrust
    C. Positive supporting reaction
    D. Neck righting

14. What do the initials MBO stand for?
    A. Management, bettered, outcomes
    B. Manager, believed, outcomes
    C. Management, by, objective
    D. Manager, bought, outcomes

15. When an elderly patient is ready for discharge from an acute hospital, equipment for home must be considered. Medicare covers durable medical equipment, which is defined as all of the following *except*:
    A. Can withstand repeated use
    B. The cost is set by Medicare
    C. Is primarily for medical purposes
    D. Is not useful in absence of illness or injury

16. Culture can have an impact on behavior. The development of suspiciousness and paranoid ideas is *most* commonly found in which of the following populations?
    A. Immigrants
    B. African-Americans
    C. Caucasians
    D. Native Americans

who exhibits poor integration of primitive reflexes with
‐body movements. What would be the *best* intervention

bows from a prone position
ye ROM
nd coordination

‐iagonal patterns, manual contacts, and distinct verbal and tactile

B. Proprioceptive neuromuscular facilitation (PNF)
C. Brunnstrom
D. Bobath

19. The Directive Group was developed by Kathy Kaplan. It may be described as all of the fol-
lowing *except*:
A. It is based on the model of human occupation
B. It is designed for higher functioning patients
C. Group leaders are active and supportive
D. Groups are often co-led

20. The president of AOTA is:
A. Elected by the representative assembly
B. Elected by the AOTA membership
C. Appointed by AOTA executive director
D. Last year's vice president

21. How many degrees of freedom of motion are available at the hip joint?
A. 1
B. 2
C. 3
D. 4

22. Which of the following statements is *not* true about delirium?
A. Delirium is a disease
B. Mood, perception, and behavior may be abnormal
C. Causes include CNS disease, systemic disease, intoxication, or withdrawal from substances
D. The neuroanatomical area effected is the reticular formation

23. Which of the following activities is the *best* choice for a client with multiple personality dis-
order whose goal is to increase her self-understanding and to express her feelings?
A. Horticulture
B. Arts and crafts
C. Sports
D. Art therapy

24. The collateral ligaments of the MP joints are taut in:
    A. Flexion
    B. Extension
    C. Abduction
    D. Adduction

25. The muscular pad created by intrinsic muscles to the fifth digit is known as the:
    A. Thenar eminence
    B. Hypothenar eminence
    C. Palmar crease
    D. Palmar arch

26. A patient diagnosed with Alzheimer's disease is about to be discharged to his home. A critical occupational therapy goal at this time should include:
    A. Increase level of activity
    B. Education of client
    C. Education of caregiver
    D. Increase memory aids

27. The *most* important area of occupational therapy intervention for a person with LE, above knee amputation is:
    A. Adaptive equipment assessment
    B. Instruction in donning and doffing the prosthetic device
    C. Gait training
    D. Teaching the client skin inspection of the stump

28. Uniform Terminology includes:
    A. Occupational performance areas and occupational performance components
    B. Definitions of current frames of reference
    C. Suggestions for documentation methods including SOAP and POMR
    D. Budget guidelines for OT departments

29. What nerve passes through the carpal tunnel?
    A. Median
    B. Ulnar
    C. Radial
    D. Musculocutaneous

30. The end feel is the sensation transmitted to the therapist's hands at the extreme end of PROM and indicates the structures that limit joint movement. A soft end feel is:
    A. Firm, from a soft tissue stretch
    B. Abrupt, with a hard stop to the movement
    C. Soft, from a soft tissue opposition
    D. Capsular, like stretching a piece of leather

31. Which of the following causes of dementia is reversible?
    A. Alzheimer's
    B. Vascular disease
    C. AIDS
    D. Depression

32. The accreditation committee of AOTA is responsible for the approval of:
    A. Certification of COTAs and the registration of OTRs
    B. Occupational therapy educational programs
    C. Licensure in states
    D. Policies in AOTA

Use the following information to answer questions 33 and 34: Another occupational therapist has told you during lunch that she is really behind in her billable units for the week so she is going to bill patients for the time this week and make up for it next week.

33. This breaks what section of the AOTA code of ethics?
    A. Principle 1, beneficence
    B. Principle 2, autonomy, privacy, and confidentiality
    C. Principle 5, veracity
    D. Principle 6, fidelity and veracity

34. The *best* response to this situation is:
    A. Notify the billing department that false billing has occurred
    B. Notify the area coordinator that there is a problem in the department
    C. Speak to the therapist privately and tell her that this is unethical
    D. Report the unethical behavior to the ethics committee of AOTA

35. When evaluating a client with an orthopedic condition, which frame of reference is *best*?
    A. Sensory motor
    B. Cognitive
    C. Developmental
    D. Biomechanical

36. The *best* group activity designed specifically for the chronically mentally ill patient who has difficulty with motor planning, verbalization, and eye contact is:
    A. Tennis
    B. Basketball
    C. Walking
    D. Parachute games

37. A homonymous hemianopsia is a loss of visual field secondary to a CVA. What would be the visual loss for a right CVA?
    A. Right nasal side and temporal of both the right and left eyes
    B. Right nasal side of right eye only
    C. Left nasal side of right eye and left temporal side of left eye
    D. Left nasal side of left eye only

38. If a client's UE is extremely difficult to move and PROM is impos
    A. Athetoid
    B. Flaccid
    C. Spastic
    D. Ataxic

39. The OTR shows a group of children several items on a table. Wnic
    eyes, the OTR removes one item. The children open their eyes and guess whicn n
    ing. Which of the following goals is *most* developed by the children?
    A. Increase eye-hand coordination
    B. Increase bilateral integration
    C. Increase form constancy
    D. Increase visual memory

40. Social smiling in infancy can be elicited by the mother at what age?
    A. 1 to 2 weeks
    B. 2 to 4 weeks
    C. 4 to 8 weeks
    D. 16 weeks

41. Medicare will pay for all of the following *except*:
    A. Trapeze
    B. Splints
    C. Bedside commode
    D. Grab bars

42. An adult with schizophrenia can be diagnosed from all of the following symptoms *except*:
    A. Social dysfunction
    B. Delusions
    C. Disorganized speech
    D. Substance abuse

43. The World Federation of Occupational Therapists (WFOT) is:
    A. Composed of NBCOT-registered OTs who work overseas
    B. Managed by AOTA
    C. Composed of OTs from around the world
    D. Part of your membership from AOTA

44. Facilitation of patient acceptance of an amputation is often addressed by occupational therapy.
    What is the *most* important area addressed to encourage acceptance of the prosthetic device?
    A. Patient's acceptance of new body image
    B. Patient's ability to deny or express anger
    C. Patient's ability to accept dependence
    D. Patient's ability to use adaptive equipment with the prosthetic device

se the following information to answer questions 45 and 46: A parent complains to the OTR at her 6-year-old child does not listen to her when she tells him to be quiet in church and stop bothering other people.

45. The OTR recognizes the child's behavior as:
A. Negativism
B. Symbolization
C. Egocentrism
D. Imminent justice

46. The *best* response the OTR could give to the mother is:
A. Ignore the child's behavior
B. Educate the parents to normal development
C. Talk to the child about his behavior
D. To redirect the child's attention to something else

47. The most common hallucination for patients with schizophrenia is:
A. Visual
B. Auditory
C. Tactile
D. Olfactory

48. The *best* example of an activity that uses Allen's cognitive disability frame of reference is:
A. Leather lacing a wallet
B. Discussion group
C. Movement or dance therapy
D. Draw a person

49. Medicare will pay for durable medical equipment if it meets the criteria and is ordered by a physician. A physician's order must include all of the following *except*:
A. Estimated cost
B. Diagnosis
C. Prognosis
D. Reason for need

50. An OTR is performing a COTE assessment on a 15-year-old male patient who is feeling depressed. He stops his activity after 2 to 3 minutes and tells the therapist that he is "too tired" to continue. The OTR hypothesizes that he has difficulty with:
A. Reality orientation
B. Initiating activity
C. Responsibility
D. Problem solving

Section Eight

51. An OTR consulting to a long-term care facility should do all of the following *except*:
A. Provide input on selection of forms and the documentation process
B. Keep activity personnel appraised of changes in regulations
C. Suggest ways staff can do physical therapy activities to cover the lack of PTs
D. Advise on enhancement of group dynamics and resident involvement

2. Universal precautions help prevent transmission of HIV and Hepatitis B. The body fluids that universal precautions applies to include:
   A. Blood and other fluids containing blood
   B. Feces and urine
   C. Sweat
   D. Tears

3. A teenage girl with muscular dystrophy wants to apply her own make-up. As her occupational therapist you recommend all of the following *except*:
   A. Prop elbow on the table to save energy
   B. Groom in phases with rest breaks
   C. Take a long shower before starting
   D. Enlarge the handles on the make-up items

4. At 40 weeks of age, a child is approximately capable of all of the following *except*:
   A. Sitting alone
   B. Creeping
   C. Ability to say one word
   D. Feeling shame

5. JCAHO accredits health care facilities. What do the initials stand for?
   A. Joint Commission on Accreditation of Healthcare Organizations
   B. Joint Committee for Accreditation of Hospital Operations
   C. Joint Consensus on Accreditation of Healthcare Operations
   D. Joint Caregivers for Accreditation of Hospital Organization

6. In a stressful situation, the difference between the function of the sympathetic and parasympathetic branches of the autonomic nervous system is all of the following *except*:
   A. Increased heart rate and force of contraction
   B. Pupils of the eyes dilate
   C. Increased sweat and secretions of the salivary gland
   D. Contract the pupils of the eye

7. Persons with AIDS are prone to opportunistic diseases. Which of the following is *not* likely to be seen in a person with AIDS?
   A. Amyotrophic lateral sclerosis
   B. Kaposi's sarcoma
   C. Pneumocystic carinii pneumonia
   D. Toxoplasmosis

8. The science of workplace design is called:
   A. Workspace planning
   B. Accessibility planning
   C. Work hardening
   D. Ergonomics

9. A client who wants to use a computer but only has gross motor hand movement would use what type of input device?
   A. Standard keyboard
   B. Expanded keyboard
   C. Joystick
   D. Single switch

10. During a home visit with a young mother who recently injured herself in a fall, you overhear her husband hitting their son repeatedly upstairs. Your client begins to cry and suddenly appears frightened. She asks you to leave because she does not want her husband to see you. What should you do?
    A. Leave as you are told
    B. Ignore the incident until further proof
    C. Run upstairs to stop the beating
    D. Secure the safety of the patient and report the abuse to authorities

11. Chronic obstructive pulmonary disease (COPD) refers to all diseases that cause irreversible damage to the lungs. For the patient with COPD, all of the following activities are consistently difficult *except*:
    A. Decision making
    B. Eating
    C. Speaking
    D. Exercise

12. A young healthy adult below age 40 will have blood pressure of less than:
    A. 120/80
    B. 130/90
    C. 140/80
    D. 140/90

13. A child must be able to identify body positioning in space and realize the course of movement to change his or her position to another position. This awareness of space direction will directly affect which of the following?
    A. Sorting one body part to another
    B. Reading and writing from left to right
    C. Picking an object out against a background
    D. Drawing a person

14. When speaking to a person with hearing impairment, the OTR should do all of the following *except*:
    A. Keep hands away from your face
    B. Speak slower
    C. Talk face to face
    D. Get the person's attention before starting to speak

15. Tracing one's body on a sheet of paper is *most* useful with what typ/
    A. Major depression
    B. Eating disorder
    C. Schizophrenia, paranoid type
    D. Bipolar, manic phase

16. Which of the following activities is the *best* initial choice for a patient in an acute paranoid state?
    A. Cooking group
    B. Reading a newspaper
    C. Organizing a daily schedule
    D. Arts and crafts

17. Which is *not* true of multiple sclerosis?
    A. It is a slowly progressive disease of the central nervous system
    B. It is characterized by demyelination of nerves
    C. Symptoms have exacerbations and remissions
    D. The onset of the disease is most common between ages 3 to 8

18. What is the *best* treatment for an adult with a head injury at Rancho Los Amigos level I or II?
    A. Community re-entry activities
    B. A functional task such as making a sandwich
    C. A simple task such as painting a birdhouse with one color
    D. PROM and sensory stimulation

19. Vegetative signs in depression include all of the following *except*:
    A. Psychomotor retardation
    B. Obsessive ruminations
    C. Weight loss
    D. Abnormal menses

20. Which of the following statements is *not* true regarding ECT treatments?
    A. Commonly used for major depressive disorder
    B. Patient experiences no movement during treatment
    C. Appearance of gooseflesh is noted
    D. A secondary stimulus may be needed to induce a seizure

21. What age group has a normal pulse rate of 115 to 130 beats per minute?
    A. First year after birth
    B. Childhood years
    C. Adult years
    D. Later years

22. Can an adult be first diagnosed with mental retardation?
    A. Yes, but only if there is a previously history of mental retardation from birth
    B. Yes, even without a history of mental retardation
    C. Yes, but only if another psychiatric diagnosis can be found
    D. No, only children can be diagnosed with mental retardation

23. Rehabilitative or educational technologies include all of the following *except*:
    A. Prosthesis
    B. Cognitive rehabilitation software
    C. Biofeedback
    D. Functional electrical stimulation

24. Which of the following OT groups is the *best* choice for a patient who is abusing substances and has a poor self-concept?
    A. Arts and crafts
    B. Cooking
    C. Shopping
    D. Life management

25. Activities such as slow, rhythmic rocking; deep breathing; and mental imagery are relevant choices for what type of OT group?
    A. Leisure skills
    B. Value clarification
    C. Stress management
    D. Weight management

26. Good skin techniques are important for children with spina bifida. These techniques include all of the following *except*:
    A. Thick and deep padding
    B. Check skin for pressure sores
    C. Change positions frequently
    D. Avoid tight fitting clothes

27. All of the following counseling techniques are appropriate to use with a newly admitted patient *except*:
    A. Confrontation
    B. Empathy
    C. Concreteness
    D. Respect

28. A person with restricted ROM throughout the UE would *best* benefit from what adaptive equipment?
    A. Extended or lengthened handles of eating utensils
    B. Rocker knife
    C. Built-up handles
    D. Spill-proof cup

29. Which of the following is *not* true of attention deficit disorder?
    A. More boys are affected than girls
    B. Children are of average or above average intelligence
    C. Children have fair to good problem solving
    D. Symptoms might include impulsiveness and hyperactivity

30. In the elderly, age-related changes such as gait, postural instability, decreased vision, decreased hearing, and forgetfulness all increase the risk of what?
   A. Drug dependence
   B. Falls
   C. Loneliness
   D. Entering a nursing home

31. What defense is your patient using when he tells you he sent his wife roses after a physical fight with her?
   A. Projection
   B. Undoing
   C. Splitting
   D. Passive-aggressive

32. Joint protection techniques include all of the following *except*:
   A. Maintain joints in correct position
   B. Use hands instead of shoulders
   C. Bend hips and knees but keep back straight
   D. Distribute load over two of more joints

33. When is anxiety considered pathological?
   A. When intensity does not match the situation
   B. When it accompanies something new
   C. When considering one's identity
   D. When facing an illness

34. A fracture in a diseased or weakened bone that has been subjected to a normal strain is called:
   A. Greenstick fracture
   B. Pathological fracture
   C. Compound fracture
   D. Comminuted fracture

35. How should flammable arts and craft supplies such as paint, stain, cleaners, and thinners be stored in the OT clinic?
   A. In a locked closet
   B. In an open area, supervised by staff
   C. In a ventilated metal cabinet
   D. In a room with a sink and water

36. Ankylosing spondylitis can result in a rigid spinal column with flexion and rotation of the trunk severely restricted. What ADL tasks would be *most* difficult for this patient?
   A. Bathing
   B. Donning shoes and socks
   C. Feeding self
   D. Meal preparation

37. What type of disease is rheumatoid arthritis?
    A. A degenerative joint disease
    B. An inflammatory joint disease
    C. A disease seen only in the elderly population
    D. A joint disease that affects the large diarthrodial joints only

38. A 46-year-old male comes to you complaining of diffuse left elbow pain. His elbow becomes stiff when he picks things up with his left hand and the pain in his left hand increases. What frame of reference would you use to treat his lateral epicondylitis?
    A. Model of human occupation
    B. Acquisitional
    C. Biomechanical
    D. Developmental

39. Why is it important to ask a patient about his or her hobbies, lifestyle, and occupations in relationship to hand use?
    A. To help establish patient rapport
    B. A repetitive pattern of use may become apparent
    C. To see if the patient has a good balance of activities in his or her life
    D. To suggest a job change before you examine the hand

40. Which evaluation is *best* to measure developmental skills in a pediatric population?
    A. Southern California Sensory Integration Tests (SCSIT)
    B. Motor Free Visual Perception Test (MVPT)
    C. Miller Assessment for Preschoolers (MAP)
    D. Play Skills Inventory

41. CHAMPUS is:
    A. A health insurance for people in the military services
    B. A program of AOTA
    C. Special research of OTs and primates
    D. A mouthpiece to use on a computer

42. Medicare Part B is:
    A. Supplementary medical insurance
    B. Available to all U. S. citizens
    C. Free to those age 65 and over
    D. Not available to those people with end stage renal disease

43. When a patient falls in the clinic, the first thing that should be done after ensuring the patient's safety and well-being is:
    A. File an incident report following the facility's policies
    B. Call the family and let them know
    C. Take the patient's temperature and blood pressure
    D. Notify the next shift of the problem

44. Evaluating a patient begins:
    A. As soon as the patient walks (or is wheeled) into the clinic
    B. When performing AROM to observe limitations
    C. While reading the medical referral
    D. While making small talk with the patient prior to testing PROM

45. Precautions for dysphasia patients include all of the following *except*:
    A. After feeding, patient should remain upright for 20 minutes to prevent aspiration
    B. If food remains in the mouth after feeding, have patient wash it down with a drink
    C. Do not schedule eating sessions after strenuous activity
    D. Do not use foods with nuts, fibers, or extreme spices that are difficult to chew

46. While conducting an ADL evaluation, your patient with schizophrenia conveys very little information and tends to respond vaguely to your questions. This speech disturbance is known as:
    A. Dysarthria
    B. Pressured speech
    C. Poverty of speech
    D. Poverty of content of speech

47. Which is *not* one of the general cognitive changes considered to be part of the normal aging process?
    A. Loss of brain cells
    B. Impaired thought processes
    C. Temporary decrease in mental function decrease following an acute illness
    D. Ability to solve practical problems in daily living

48. All of the following are effective in reducing hand edema for the post surgery client *except*:
    A. Cold, wet packs
    B. Massage
    C. Elevation
    D. Isotoner brand gloves

49. What type of spoon should be used to feed a child with reflex biting?
    A. A traditional teaspoon
    B. A traditional soup spoon
    C. A narrow, shallow, plastic spoon
    D. A square-shaped spade spoon

50. While working with a patient who is post myocardial infarction, activities should be stopped when all of the following signs are present *except*:
    A. Dyspnea
    B. Palpitations
    C. Pulse between 95 to 110
    D. Glassy stare

Section Nine

1. Splinting of the wrist for the treatment of carpal tunnel syndrome should be static to prevent movement. At which position should the wrist be?
   A. 10° to 20° extension
   B. 10° to 20° flexion
   C. 5° ulnarly deviated
   D. 30° flexion

2. Prism glasses are ideal for:
   A. Patients with a halo or confined flat in bed
   B. Magnifying book pages
   C. Improving colors for low vision clients
   D. Not spilling drinks, when patients have hand tremors

3. A child with spastic cerebral palsy has scissor gait. This means the hip muscles are:
   A. In flexion
   B. In abduction
   C. Internally rotated
   D. Externally rotated

4. Caffeine withdrawal includes all of the following *except*:
   A. Hallucinations
   B. Nervousness
   C. Insomnia
   D. Headache

5. An OTR is leading a coping skills group for people with AIDS. Which of the following is inappropriate for the OTR to tell clients during the group?
   A. Feeling guilt is common
   B. Homosexuals should not "come out" to their families at this time
   C. Discussion of terminal care
   D. Practice of safe sex is necessary

6. You are doing tactile stimulation with a group of three children. The children are lying on a mat and you are rolling a large ball over them. They like the feeling and ask you to do it again. What is the *best* response to the request?
   A. Say no, explain that they have had enough
   B. Repeat the activity, this time putting more pressure on the ball
   C. Say it is time to try something new
   D. Try bouncing the ball over them

7. Which of the following is *not* true about anorexia nervosa?
   A. The essential feature is binge eating
   B. Patients have a tendency toward perfectionism
   C. Body image is distorted
   D. Starvation and suicide are common causes of death

8. In what position should the neck be splinted for a pediatric patient with burns?
   A. 10° hyperextension
   B. 10° flexion
   C. Flexion, as much as possible
   D. 0° neutral

9. A hyperactive gag reflex may be normalized by:
   A. Icing the lips and having the patient say "OOO."
   B. Offering resistance to opening the jaw
   C. Walking a tongue depressor toward the back of the tongue
   D. Sucking through a 6-inch straw and gradually increasing the straw length

10. If a patient slightly cuts his finger while cutting vegetables in the ADL kitchen, the OTR should follow universal precautions and then:
    A. Call a medical emergency
    B. Hand the patient a gauze and ask him to apply pressure to the cut
    C. Call his nurse to the kitchen
    D. Call the OT supervisor for assistance

11. A patient with bilateral proximal UE weakness would benefit from what type of equipment while self-feeding?
    A. Enlarged handles on utensils
    B. Scoop dish
    C. Rocker knife
    D. Mobile arm supports

12. All of the following conditions may lead to child abuse and neglect *except*:
    A. Low self-esteem of the parent(s)
    B. Mothers in their 20s
    C. Frustration with the child's toilet training
    D. Lack of support for family

13. All of the following statements regarding HIV and AIDS are true *except*:
    A. Most infections secondary to HIV involve the central nervous system
    B. Prozac may be prescribed to deal with depression secondary to HIV
    C. No person should be given an HIV test without prior consent or knowledge
    D. HIV is a DNA retrovirus

14. Your patient is a young child with significant hearing loss due to a lesion in the middle ear. Which of the following areas might be a strength?
    A. Bilateral coordination
    B. Visual concentration
    C. Self-perception
    D. Play skills

15. In high velocity head injuries a cranial nerve is commonly damaged. The results are a decrease in the sense to smell and therefore a decrease in appetite. What cranial nerve is this?
   A. I
   B. III
   C. IV
   D. V

16. A bowel program for the patient with a spinal cord injury includes all of the following *except*:
   A. Timing and a regular schedule
   B. Hot oral intake
   C. Suppository or digital stimulation
   D. Convenient time in patient's schedule

17. In order to achieve the mechanical advantage of a stand pivot transfer, the client must first:
   A. Unlock the wheelchair
   B. Angle the wheelchair 90° to the transfer location
   C. Scoot forward in the chair
   D. Do nothing, but the person providing the transfer must stand in front of the client with feet 30 cm apart

18. When comparing developmental norms between children with sight and children without sight, which is true concerning motor development?
   A. There is no difference
   B. Children who are blind develop more rapidly
   C. Children who are blind have motor delays
   D. Children who have sight have motor delays

19. Which of the following statements is *not* true concerning patients with chronic pain?
   A. Depression is frequent
   B. ADL activities may be avoided by the patient
   C. Pain is real to the patient
   D. Job performance is maintained

20. Which of the following goals would address poor coordination and atypical postures in a child with failure to thrive?
   A. Develop play skills
   B. Increase response to stimuli to normal range
   C. Increase gross motor to normal range
   D. Increase independence in ADLs

21. Factors used to indicate the severity of head injury and estimate the outcome include all of the following *except*:
   A. Glasgow Coma Scale
   B. Post traumatic amnesia
   C. Galvestine Orientation and Amnesia Test
   D. Assessment of tone and posturing using MMT

22. Dantrium (dantrolene) is often given to patients with spinal cord injuries to decrease spasticity. A side effect of this medication might include:
    A. Seizures
    B. Liver toxicity hepatitis
    C. Hallucinations
    D. Decreased blood pressure

23. Energy conservation techniques include all of the following *except*:
    A. Sit to work
    B. Limit amount of work
    C. Organize storage
    D. Plan one day at a time

24. An adolescent with a spinal cord injury is refusing to cooperate in the formal occupational therapy assessment at admission. What is the *best* option for the OTR?
    A. Administer a different assessment
    B. Use informal methods at first
    C. Discontinue the assessment and wait until the patient is more cooperative
    D. Tell the teenager that you will have to tell his parents

25. Which of the following patients would best benefit from a wheelchair with removable arms?
    A. The head injured client who might get confused by arm rests
    B. The elder patient with ataxia who needs to get to the tub or sink
    C. The patient with T4 spinal cord lesion who wants to use a transfer board
    D. The patient with Alzheimer's disease who can reach items dropped

26. The general rule regarding a person using alcohol after a severe head injury is:
    A. 4 to 6 weeks post injury
    B. Limit of one drink per day
    C. 2 years post injury
    D. Never drink again

27. The most common complaint of the patient with a spinal cord injury is:
    A. Depression
    B. Spasticity
    C. Fatigue
    D. Bladder control

28. Medications to reduce seizures in patients with head injuries might produce what side effect?
    A. Increase in emotional depression
    B. Increase in agitation
    C. Decrease in speech due to dry mouth
    D. Decrease in cognitive performance

29. Which of the following terms *best* describes a child who may incur developmental delays, disorders, or deficits because of factors occurring before, during, or after birth?
    A. Mental retardation
    B. High-risk infant
    C. Failure to thrive
    D. Learning disabilities

30. Which of the following is *not* characteristic of normal adolescence?
    A. Acting out behavior
    B. Occasional delinquent acts
    C. Episodes of depression
    D. Increased closeness to siblings and parents

31. According to Anne Mosey, what term describes social structure, values, norms, and expectations shared by people?
    A. Human environment
    B. Social environment
    C. Nonhuman environment
    D. Cultural environment

32. Who among the following is *not* responsible for OT group treatment approaches?
    A. Gail Fidler
    B. Irvin Yalom
    C. Anne Mosey
    D. Mildred Ross

33. According to Uniform Terminology, all of the following OT goals are appropriate to the motor component of a leather working task *except*:
    A. Increase bilateral coordination
    B. Increase eye-hand coordination
    C. Increase organization
    D. Increase hand strength

34. When taking patients with mental health disabilities outside in the sun, the OTR needs to remember that patients on psychotropic medications:
    A. Burn easily
    B. Are sensitive to light
    C. Need to drink a lot of water
    D. Get muscle cramps easily

Use the following information to answer questions 35 and 36: Heterotrophic ossification can be a common medical condition of patients in rehabilitation programs.

35. People with all of the following may experience heterotrophic ossification *except*:
    A. Head injury
    B. Spinal cord injury
    C. Burns
    D. Multiple sclerosis

36. The most common site of heterotrophic ossification is the:
    A. Elbow
    B. Finger
    C. Hip
    D. Shoulder

37. Allen's Cognitive Levels (ACL) provide a therapist with information on what could be expected of a patient at different levels. What activity would be *best* for a person with an ACL score of 1?
    A. Community activities such as shopping for hair care products
    B. Task activities such as lacing a wallet
    C. ADL activities such as brushing one's teeth
    D. Simple activity such as listening to music in the patient's room

38. The leading cause of death for a person with a spinal cord injury is:
    A. Cardiovascular problems
    B. Respiratory problems
    C. Urinary tract infections
    D. Spasticity

39. Quality assurance is all of the following *except*:
    A. Supported by AOTA
    B. No longer optional in hospitals
    C. In constant development and continuous in monitoring
    D. Required even in public school systems

40. The lateral curvature of the spine is:
    A. Kyphosis
    B. Spina bifida
    C. Scoliosis
    D. Rickets

41. Sacs of fluid located in areas of friction, especially in joints, are called:
    A. Bursae
    B. Fascia
    C. Ligaments
    D. Tendons

42. Positioning of a patient who is bedbound for an extended time should include all of the following *except*:
    A. Knees lifted by a pillow while supine
    B. One pillow under head while supine
    C. Frequent position changes
    D. No pillow under head, but one under knees while supine

...ak your language is resistive and frightened to transfer from the bed ...rapy. What is the occupational therapist's *best* approach?

...firm "Yes you can, I will help you"

...transfer the patient before you come up

...r with another therapist

...e patient and transfer him while making eye contact

...a mastectomy and undergoing chemotherapy will have many issues in occupational therapy including both physical and psychosocial rehabilitation. All of the following are appropriate *except*:

A. If the patient initiates the questions first, the therapist can answer questions about prognosis, treatments available for cancer, and pain medications

B. Teach energy conservation and work simplification techniques

C. Use counseling skills to address body issues and role changes

D. Provide strengthening exercises and share MMT results with patient

45. Quality assurance (QA) requires the development of indicators as variables that indicate quality care of the patient. All of the following would be appropriate occupational therapy indicators in a mental health service *except*:

A. Occupational therapy assessment initiated within 24 hours of admission

B. QA plan will be monitored monthly

C. Patient involvement in goal setting is indicated by patient signature on OT treatment plan

D. Safety hazards are reported during the shift in which they are discovered

46. Early intervention services for children from birth to 3 years old can be remedial or preventive to children with disabilities. Which of the following is *not* true about this approach?

A. Play activities activate neurons

B. Critical periods for brain development extend from early childhood to middle childhood

C. The brain of a young child is known to be highly plastic

D. Cognitive, language, motor, perceptual, and emotional development are interdependent

Use the following information to answer questions 47 and 48: A 65-year-old widowed woman you are treating for an acute exacerbation of arthritis has been hinting around that she is having problems at home. Sensing that she does not want to talk about her problems in an open area you ask her to meet with you in your office so you can have a private moment to speak with her. She tells you that she is "uncomfortable having sex with her new boyfriend." After talking further with her, she has identified joint pain as the problem.

47. Which of the following is crucial to the OTR's ability to provide effective sexual counseling to this client or any other?

A. Extensive awareness of anatomy and physiology

B. Awareness of personal attitudes about sexuality, sex roles, and sexual preferences

C. Details about the client's sexual history

D. The referral process to a sex therapist

48. What is the *best* advice to give to this client at this time?
    A. The client should ask the boyfriend to give up sex until she is in remission
    B. Educate and encourage the client to try different sexual positions to reduce joint pain
    C. Suggest the couple try other romantic activities instead of sex until she feels better
    D. Tell the client that she should slow down and act her age

49. Which of the following is *not* true regarding sensory stimulation treatment for children with mental retardation?
    A. Helps to increase level of arousal
    B. Increases ability to focus attention
    C. Eliminates stereotyped behaviors
    D. Finding appropriate level of stimulation is important to success

50. A child has usually established hand preference by what age?
    A. 2
    B. 5
    C. 7
    D. 9

Chapter Six
Answers and Explanations

SECTION ONE

1. Answer: D
When a patient with a spinal cord injury complains of dizziness, nausea, and is losing consciousness while standing in a standing box, the patient is experiencing postural hypotension. Recline him immediately and get medical assistance if symptoms persist.

2. Answer: B
Work tolerance is a performance skill. A, C, and D are performance components of Uniform Terminology.

3. Answer: A
Project level play is for children under 8 years old. B, C, and D are typical of 8-year-olds.

4. Answer: D
The occupational therapist does not have to be hospital affiliated; however, A, B, and C are required for Medicare reimbursement.

5. Answer: C
Inflammation of the forearm musculature (ECRB, ECRL, EDC) may result in tennis elbow.

6. Answer: B
Sublimation is the healthy and acceptable rechanneling of the libidinal and aggressive drives into constructive activity. This defense was identified by Anna Freud and remains a basic component to occupational therapy activity. Acting out is often negative and externalizes an unresolved conflict. Identification is a term that incorporates the characteristics of another onto oneself. Regression is going backwards to an earlier stage of development.

7. Answer: A
Uniform Terminology does not provide any information about fees. B, C, and D are all true of Uniform Terminology.

8. Answer: D
An entry-level COTA is defined as a COTA with less than 1 year of experience. The COTA's work must be supervised by an OTR for the first year.

9. Answer: D
Connective tissue disease is not associated with depression, dementia, or psychosis, while Parkinson's, Huntington's, and Wilson's diseases are associated with them.

10. Answer: D

The anterior longitudinal ligament limits extension to protect the vertebral column from excess extension. The posterior longitudinal ligament protects the spine in flexion. Ligamentum flavum is too small and supraspinatus is a muscle.

11. Answer: D

Abnormal tone, delayed or exaggerated reflexes, and abnormal motor development are all signs of cerebral palsy.

12. Answer: B

Emotional flight is dominated by the sympathetic nervous system.

13. Answer: C

Direct services means the OTR is providing face-to-face treatment services.

14. Answer: A

Labile describes abrupt and rapid emotional changes. Anhedonia is the loss of interest and withdrawal from pleasurable activities. Inappropriate affect refers to a mismatch between an emotion and the idea, thought, or speech expressed. Euphoric is the intense feeling of grandeur or happiness.

15. Answer: C

Atrophy is not a symptom of spasticity, while A, B, and D are.

16. Answer: D

An OTR, self-employed, must carry individual coverage.

17. Answer: C

Treatment documentation should not include the patient's bill balance. A, B, and D should be included.

18. Answer: B

The patient will need a dressing stick, sock aid, longhandled shoe horn, bath sponge, and reacher for some time after discharge to achieve independence. A tea cart is not essential as the patient could slide items on the counter. A tub seat is optional but only if the patient is not safe in the tub. The commode should not be necessary as most patients at discharge no longer need one; however, a bedside urinal would be adequate if needed.

19. Answer: C

Tenodesis action is enhanced by shortening the flexor tendons.

20. Answer: C

Licensure is a state responsibility; registration and certification are AOTA.

21. Answer: B

Overall objective, derived goals, and key participants are unique to MBO plans.

22. Answer: C

Systematic desensitization is an effective treatment for persons with anxiety disorders. A behavioral technique that uses relaxation with an anxiety-producing stimulus will diminish the anxiety response. Habilitation refers to enabling the person to learn a skill he or she has never learned. Extinction is a behavioral approach used to discourage a behavior by ignoring it and reinforcing acceptable ones. Token economy is a reward for a desired behavior.

23. Answer: B

Components of the flexor synergy include scapular adduction, elevation, shoulder abduction, and external rotation.

24. Answer: B

Components of the flexor synergy include elbow flexion and forearm supination.

25. Answer: B

Outpatient services are covered as part of an office visit to a physician. A, C, and D are not true.

26. Answer: A

Family abuse toward people with disabilities is a significant problem that is often under reported. Supportive questions may clarify this situation and encourage the patient to share her concerns. Dysphagia can be the result of attempted strangulation. B and C are appropriate to typical treatment. D is a weak choice because it ignores the patient's issues.

27. Answer: C

These are defining aspects of frame of reference. A paradigm is a guiding premise and theory which leads to the organization of knowledge, such as the OT profession. A model is a profession's philosophical assumption, ethics, foundation, and domain of concern. Therapeutic use of self is the manner in which the therapist views him- or herself and the impact on one's clients.

28. Answer: C

The cerebellum plays a role in the excitation of gamma motor neurons which innervate intrafusal fibers within muscles. Damage to the cerebellum causes a decrease in the excitation of gamma motor neurons which, in turn, leads to a decrease in the sensitivity of the muscle spindles. A decrease in muscle tone results. Hypertonia is an increase in tone. Both rigidity and spasticity are examples of hypertonia.

29. Answer: D

A person with a total knee replacement must learn to bend the knee to increase range of motion. A, B, and C would discourage movement at the knee and therefore are inappropriate.

30. Answer: D

The ventral root carries motor information from the motor cortex out to the muscles. Efferent projections are motor in nature and carry output from a neural structure. Afferent projections are sensory in nature and carry input to a neural structure such as a sensory receptor to the somatosensory lobe.

31. Answer: A

According to Patricia Parmelee, associate director of research at the Philadelphia Geriatric Center, depression is closely linked with physical illness and disability when it causes functional loss. B, C, and D are possible factors in the contribution of depression, however, they do not always lead to depression. Persons experiencing depression in later life seem to be more responsive to treatment.

32. Answer: B

Three times the oxygen of rest is consumed in self-care activities. Climbing stairs is 5 METs and walking fast is 7 METs.

33. Answer: A

Fever is usually an indicator of infection. B, C, and D are indicators of cardiac dysfunction.

34. Answer: C

The patient must be free of chest pain and would stop exercising at the first sign of pain. B and D are important to address after pain. The patient may need reassurance to the safety of exercise and how he or she is to be monitored. A patient's depression may last up to 6 months.

35. Answer: A

Education begins at phase 1 including vocational, family, and sexual issues. Phase 2 continues education and MET level 5 activities. At this level the occupational therapist begins to discuss return to work and a possible job site evaluation. Phase 3 and outpatient usually coincide.

36. Answer: D

Anxiety and stress are issues of first priority for most patients. Learning to decrease these symptoms is the priority. A, B, and C are also very important but come next in line once the patient is feeling more control.

37. Answer: B

The static/tonic reflex is initiated by a slow stretch of a muscle. This causes stimulation of motor units in the muscle to create resistance. The phasic/dynamic stretch reflex is elicited by rapid muscle stretch and opposes sudden changes in muscle length. The inverse stretch reflex causes a muscle to relax once the maximum tension is reached. The withdrawal/flexor reflex is a response generally initiated by pain or tissue damage. Flexion or withdrawal of the affected body part then occurs.

38. Answer: D

Discussion of feelings regarding suicide with empathy and respect can greatly reduce the distress of a suicidal person and decrease one's sense of isolation. Focusing exclusively about how to commit suicide without considering emotional distress can lead to "copycat" suicides. A, B, and C are all true.

39. Answer: C

During Bailey's investigation in 1990 regarding reasons for OT attrition, 29% of occupational therapists reported "burnout" as their main reason for leaving. This is a type of job stress arising from the social interaction between helper and recipient. Clinical depression is diagnosed with the presence of at least five symptoms including sadness, empty mood, anhedonia, change in sleep and/or appetite, and feelings of worthlessness. Dysthymia is a mild chronic depression lasting 2 or more years. A reaction is a response to a stimulus while a syndrome is a group of signs/symptoms that characterize a disease process.

40. Answer: D

MSDS are required to protect those exposed to workplace materials. The MSDS provide information in case of an emergency such as a child eating a piece of theraputty. MSDS are not required for personal items stored in handbags or lockers, however, safety is always first and an occupational therapist should not use personal items in clinical use without first addressing all safety issues.

41. Answer: B

Cosigning notes is not evidence of supervision. The OTR should maintain a separate log book whenever the COTA and OTR meet to review cases. C and D are incorrect.

42. Answer: A

In order to provide optimal ROM at the shoulder joint, the scapula must move 1° for every 2° of humeral movement. If this does not occur, damage may result. The head of the humerus would not have sufficient space to move in the joint.

43. Answer: D

Rett's syndrome is marked by loss of hand skills already acquired in normal development. A, B, and C do not lose hand skills and may or may not have stereotypical hand movements.

44. Answer: D

All are signs including inability to calm self, clumsiness, poor academic achievement, and delay in speech and language skills.

45. Answer: A

According to the NDT Association, abnormal muscle tone and movement affects all function including walking, speech, respiration, feeding, perception, and self-care. B, C, and D are true.

46. Answer: A

Free association is a psychoanalytic technique used by analysts with years of extensive training. All the other cognitive methods are modalities used in OT.

47. Answer: A

Developmental groups were first identified by Anne Mosey and include parallel, project, egocentric-cooperative, cooperative, and mature levels.

48. Answer: A

A muscle fiber can shorten up to one half its total length. Fusiform or strap muscles are generally longer than other types of muscle and allow the greatest ROM. Spiral and pennate muscle fibers are generally shorter and more numerous, and therefore provide greater strength.

49. Answer: C

Directive leadership means the therapist takes a more active role in group. The leader provides structure, keeps the group focused, supports members, and ensures efficient use of group time. Acute inpatient group members are usually in crisis and do not have time to reach a mature level. Directive leadership is useful in groups at a low maturity level. Facilitative leadership is effective in groups at a medium to high maturity level. Advisory leadership is effective with highly mature groups. Democratic leadership is a term that correlates with facilitative leadership.

50. Answer: B

Motor apraxia includes the awkward use of tools and poor control of mouth or oral motor control. Ideational apraxia is the misuse of a tool. Unilateral neglect means the patient does not attend to or use her affected arm. Perseveration means the patient is unable to stop movements and may continue to put food in her mouth resulting in over stuffing.

SECTION TWO

1. Answer: A

At the time of the printing of this book, physical therapy, nursing, or speech also had to service the home care patient before the OT could provide service. AOTA is working to change this policy.

2. Answer: B

Reality testing is the process of evaluating and judging one's external environment in an objective manner. Autistic thinking refers to a preoccupation with one's inner world. Magical thinking is when thoughts, words, or actions are believed to assume power. Illogical thinking is contradicting and erroneous.

3. Answer: C

Dysdiadochokinesia is impaired alternating movement. Overshooting is dysmetria, weak muscles is asthenia, and slow, twisting movements is athetosis.

4. Answer: D

All are good choices but arranging the client's environment to encourage looking to the left is best. This should be done as long as the patient is cognitively aware of the neglect. If patient is not cognitively aware of the left, visitors or other stimulus approaching from the left may scare her. Remind family and staff to announce their presence as they enter.

5. Answer: C

Subluxation itself is not painful but poor handling is. Transfers and PROM will potentially cause soft tissue damage. Pay special attention in handling and in scapula mobilization. Slings are not always helpful and should not be used 24 hours per day. A lap board may be helpful when the patient is in a wheelchair but does not address the global issue.

6. Answer: D

Fingertip prehension requires fine motor coordination. It allows one to sew, snap, or button. Palmar prehension involves three fingers for writing or eating. Lateral prehension is used when turning a key. It generally involves the thumb. Hook prehension is thumbless and is used when carrying a handle, case, or heavy object.

7. Answer: D

Two inches wider than the user is correct. One size does not fit all and too much padding or room can cause sores.

8. Answer: A

Although all activities are fine motor, age and diagnosis must be considered. B, C, and D may be too advanced for this child.

9. Answer: A

Continued passive stretching of spastic muscle may produce a sudden letting go relaxation. Claspknife phenomenon may be seen in neurological disorders of upper motor neuron lesions. Clonus is a spasmodic alteration of muscle contraction and relaxation. Rigidity is relatively constant hypertonicity. Dystonia is a tone disorder resulting in slow movement or decreased tone.

10. Answer: C

The OTR could make a memory book for the patient that includes answers to common questions like "Where am I?" Include family pictures and reality orientation information. Keep the book simple to reduce agitation and light in case the patient should throw it. Having the patient play cards or socialize with others may be too much stimulation. Doing nothing is likely to get the patient more agitated.

11. Answer: C

The difference between high and low technology is electronics.

12. Answer: C

Withdrawal is a group of symptoms that appear within hours to 1 week of abstinence from a substance. Examples include delirium, tremors, seizures, psychosis, perceptual disturbances, irritability, and gastrointestinal and sympathetic hyperactivity. Addiction refers to a behavior and physical dependence, not a symptom. Intoxication is a state of progressive deterioration ranging from exhilaration to stupefaction caused by ingesting substances. Abuse refers to a maladaptive pattern leading to clinical significant impairment or distress.

13. Answer: B

The patient's affect shows the emotional responsiveness of the patient. This may affect the data collected during the rest of the intake. Asking the patient to subtract 7 from 100 is measuring attention and knowledge. Hallucinations are disturbances in perception. Mood is a pervasive, sustained emotion reported by the patient.

14. Answer: C

All the activities encourage either community involvement or fine motor skills, but only the quilt fundraiser provides both.

15. Answer: B

The OTR should use universal precautions with all patients whether they have AIDS or not. The person with AIDS is at greater risk of catching a disease from the therapist. Staff should wash their hands before and after treatment. The OTR needs to wear a mask only if he or she has a cold. Latex gloves are only needed if there is a risk of contact with bodily fluids.

16. Answer: B

Only muscular dystrophy is an early childhood, progressive, and fatal disease due to fatty infiltration of the muscles. Post-polio syndrome is weakened musculature following poliomyelitis. Parkinson's is a slow progressive disease with onset after age 40. Multiple sclerosis is due to a demyelination of the nerves.

17. Answer: A

A premature infant is any infant born before 37 weeks.

18. Answer: C

Spinning is contraindicated for people prone to seizures. The patient may not be able to tolerate the vestibular input, thereby triggering a seizure.

19. Answer: D

Irritability, vomiting, headaches, and "setting sun" eyes are all symptoms of a malfunctioning shunt. Setting sun eyes are partially visible irises.

20. Answer: B

The anterior motor roots within the spinal cord are considered lower motor neuron. The CNS includes the brainstem, cranial nerves, and the cerebral cortex.

21. Answer: C

Occupational therapy can be paid for under both Parts A and B of Medicare.

22. Answer: C

Entry-level COTAs are required to have supervision by OTRs. All OT personnel should have supervision as needed to match their level of competence.

23. Answer: C

Utilization review is an internal management review on how resources are utilized.

24. Answer: B

Symmetrical postures predominate at 16 weeks. The startle reflex is present at birth when flexion of the extremities occur when scared. Babinski can be induced by stroking the sole of the foot and the big toe rises. This is normal until age 1 but after the toe should plantar flex. Impassive facial expressions are typical social behavior of an infant under 4 weeks of age.

25. Answer: D

Loose associations are a disturbance of thought. In severe cases, the patient may become incoherent. Blocking refers to abrupt interruptions in thinking. Perseveration refers to persistent responses often found in cognitive disorders. Flight of ideas refers to rapid thinking with shifting in ideas that are slightly connected.

26. Answer: B

A person with decreased cardiovascular endurance may benefit from aquatic therapy. A, C, and D do not indicate readiness.

27. Answer: D

Two thirds length allows full elbow motion and distributes weight over the length. This splint is a first-class lever with the pivot point or fulcrum at the wrist. The long trough distributes the weight of the hand and acts as a counterbalance. A, B, and C are too short.

28. Answer: A

Hopscotch involves motor synthesis. Answer B is tactile perception, C is cognitive problem solving, and D is visual motor synthesis.

29. Answer: D

Drawing from memory is a visual motor synthesis activity.

30. Answer: D

Wide, soft, foam-like strap is the best choice because it allows for slight fluctuations in edema. A, B, and C are less favorable.

31. Answer: B

Ability to abstract is to take an event such as a picnic and value the friendship of the people you are with as well as the food. Immediate recall is remembering information within 1 minute. Concentration is the ability to maintain attention for longer periods to complete a task. Attention is the ability of the CNS to focus on relevant stimuli while screening out irrelevant.

32. Answer: A

Compliance is enhanced if the therapist has listened to the patient's issues concerning feel and fit. B, C, and D are also valuable to apply in treatment.

33. Answer: C

Lorna Jean King believed that persons with schizophrenia have ineffective proprioceptive feedback mechanisms with an underactive vestibular regulating system. Activities should be non-cortical and pleasurable since thinking about movements tends to slow down a person. A, B, and D all require attention to the movement patterns.

34. Answer: D

The reticular formation dispersed throughout the brainstem is responsible. The basal ganglia are not located in the brainstem. Although the anterior and lateral corticospinal tracts do pass through the brainstem, they are primarily involved in motor control.

35. Answer: C

The prefrontal association circuit is involved in cognitive processing which includes attention switching. This circuit is believed to be affected in patients who are unable to control ritualistic and repetitive behaviors. The motor circuit aids in making movements automatic and coordinated and is believed to be involved in Parkinson's disorder. The oculomotor circuit plays a role in the control of eye movements and is believed to be involved in Parkinson's disorder and Huntington's disease. The limbic circuit plays a role in emotions and motivation and is believed to be involved in behaviors associated with Tourette's syndrome.

36. Answer: D

A soft splint, such as a palm protector, places joints in submaximum extension. This allows for adequate skin hygiene. Answer A is not true as options are available. Nursing can provide warm soaks. The resting hand splint is too rigid and likely painful.

37. Answer: A

Emotional stress of serious magnitude that is traumatic for almost everyone contributes to the development of PTSD. Recent research has placed greater emphasis on a person's subjective response to trauma than on the severity of the stress itself. A majority of people do not develop PTSD even when faced with overwhelming trauma.

38. Answer: A

The flexor pollicis longus originates on the body of the radius and inserts on the base of the distal phalanx of digit 1. Therefore, the muscle belly is located within the forearm and not the hand. B, C, and D all have muscle bellies located in the hand.

39. Answer: B

A child can maintain head control while supported at 2 months. At 1 month the child can move his or her head slightly while in prone. At 4 to 5 months the child can hold his or her chest off the floor when in prone.

40. Answer: C

A mature dynamic tripod grasp is typical of a 5- to 6-year-old. A less mature static tripod is used by a 3- to 4-year-old and the hand moves instead of the fingers during writing. A power grasp is used by a 1-year-old and is fisted with the wrist flexed.

41. Answer: D

ATNR and STNR are brainstem level reflexes.

42. Answer: A

Spasticity is most common and includes hyperactive deep tendon reflexes. Athetosis has varying muscle tone. Atonia is low tone, and mixed is usually spastic with athetosis.

43. Answer: D

Acceptance of one's sexual identity is a developmental task of later adolescence (18 to 22 years).

44. Answer: D

The American Spinal Cord Injury Association states that tetraplegia is the preferred term to indicate impairment or loss of motor and/or sensory function at the cervical level.

45. Answer: C

PPS has a slow onset appearing decades after the acute onset of polio or after decades of stable functioning. A, B, and D are classic signs of PPS.

46. Answer: D

Pervasive developmental disorders are distinct from schizophrenia although children with PPD may occasionally develop schizophrenia later in life.

47. Answer: C

The occupational therapist does not advise about medical procedures but may encourage the parent to ask the child's medical staff for advice.

48. Answer: D

As a consultant, you are advising the teacher and parent. Having the teenager wait until school to shave puts shaving out of the home and into an inappropriate site. Starting a shaving group would only be appropriate if everyone else in the class needed instruction but this is not the case. Currently, the young man has no male role models as everyone around him of importance is female. A male teenager volunteer could be advised to role model shaving and offer words of encouragement. An electric shaver could provide added safety.

49. Answer: D

Handling, positioning, and inhibiting techniques are NDT terms. NDT techniques can be used along with spatiotemporal frame of reference but are not foundations as are A, B, and C.

50. Answer: C

Even older adults can improve sensory integration and being active through life can facilitate this, however, basic sensory integration development is generally developed by age 8 to 10.

SECTION THREE

1. Answer: D

Cylindrical grasp is correct. All the others are types of pinch.

2. Answer: A

A neurological evaluation would always include a review of the gross motor and fine motor coordination. B, C, and D are appropriate for follow-up based on initial neurological screening.

3. Answer: C

An entry-level COTA can complete an ADL evaluation and can assist in perceptual, cognitive, and sensory motor evaluations.

4. Answer: B
Medicare Part A pays for inpatient care and does not cover outpatient visits.

5. Answer: B
The Purdue Pegboard is a test of motor skills. The Adult Activity Inventory is a leisure skills evaluation. The COTE is a behaviorally based test of general performance. The SCSIT is a pediatric test of sensory integration.

6. Answer: C
The width of the door opening should be a minimum of 32 inches.

7. Answer: B
The code of ethics cannot be altered.

8. Answer: A
Cocontraction requires both extensor and flexor muscles to be active. This means that the child must stay still, like in the game "Statue." B, C, and D are activities that work on gross motor skills and require movement.

9. Answer: C
Problem solving is considered a cognitive skill. A, B, and D are all skills included in life management and daily living.

10. Answer: A
Subjective data are any data that the patient told the therapist. Objective data are fact-based from the OT.

11. Answer: C
The acromion process is found on the posterior lateral aspect of scapula. Palpated to assess subluxation, it is also the axis of goniometry.

12. Answer: B
Boutonniere is described. Ulnar deviation is MCP deviation. Swan neck is PIP extension and DIP flexion. Intrinsic is a soft tissue test.

13. Answer: B
Safety is the first concern to prevent patient injury such as bumping or burning the involved limb. The patient must be taught compensation techniques for the sensory loss. Sensory re-education is a low priority. Spontaneous recovery may occur. Sensory loss does result in decreased motor function. The therapist should work on increasing movement considering safety first. Self-care would follow compensation techniques. The patient would need to work safely in her environment.

14. Answer: B
Job satisfaction is the number one reason why staff stay in one facility. Salaries, benefits, and education, while important, fall below satisfaction.

15. Answer: C

Although great gains have been made lately, research in OT is still considered to be in its infancy when compared to other arts and sciences. Lack of research can lead to some people thinking of occupational therapy as a second-class science. For this reason, AOTF makes research a top priority.

16. Answer: B

A client with high distractibility requires an environment with low stimuli to focus on a task. A and C are inappropriate. D is not true.

17. Answer: A

Capital expenses are major costs such as land and buildings. Supplies and equipment are direct costs if used for treatment, indirect if used as office supplies. OT staff salaries vary if direct patient care or management.

18. Answer: B

Repression is unconscious forgetting as a means of coping. Dementia refers to organic deterioration of intellectual functioning. Impaired judgment refers to the inability to assess a situation correctly and act. Regression refers to the returning to an earlier level of functioning.

19. Answer: C

Prozac has promising effects for depression, obsessive-compulsive disorder, and bulimia. Prozac is not an antipsychotic drug. All the other answers are true.

20. Answer: D

Doorknobs should be located 36 inches from the floor to allow for access for a person using a wheelchair.

21. Answer: C

Documentation must comply with regulation and laws first. Management, OT staff, and, at times, faculty can provide suggestions within the regulations.

22. Answer: D

Only NBCOT offers certification for COTAs.

23. Answer: D

The patient needs to feel the value of a vertical position and to gain head control but still needs support in the wheelchair. If tipped back, she will never be upright. This does not treat the problem. Verbal commands will only lead to frustration of both patient and therapist. Using an object can help develop strength but cannot be used continuously.

24. Answer: C

Until you speak with the mother, you will not know what the problem is. The program may be too difficult or the mother may be overwhelmed with the responsibility. When treating a child with severe disabilities, the OTR is often treating the whole family. Take time to meet with the mother privately and provide her with the support she needs.

25. Answer: B

Muscle endurance defined as how many times the muscle can contract is not determined by MMT. Resistance, ROM, and strength gains/losses can all be measured with MMT.

26. Answer: C

These are typical signs of conversion disorder. Hypochondriasis is a preoccupation with disease which is unrealistic or inaccurate of actual physical symptoms. Korsakoff's syndrome is an amnestic disorder cause by thiamine deficiency not uncommon in persons with chronic alcohol abuse or poor nutritional habits. Dissociative identity disorder is also know as multiple personality and caused by a severe traumatic event.

27. Answer: B

Weakness in the proximal hip musculature makes climbing stairs difficult for a person with myopathy. The client could lean forward to support him- or herself and continue to use distal function for A and C. Donning pants could be achieved by sitting.

28. Answer: C

The client cannot tolerate an upright position and may require a graded program in a reclining back wheelchair. Autonomic dysreflexia is a life-threatening rise in blood pressure with headache and coma. Death can occur if untreated. A pulmonary emboli is also life threatening and includes respiratory distress. Answer D is observable in some cases.

29. Answer: B

All items are important but prevention is key.

30. Answer: D

Stroke, immobilization, and MI are all at risk for DVT. Fifty percent of all people with CVA experience DVT. The lower extremities should be evaluated daily for discoloration, edema, and pain. RSD is not associated with DVT.

31. Answer: C

C6 innervates extensor carpi radialis longus and brevis. C5 has elbow flexors and limited distal function. C4 has absence of arm function.

32. Answer: B

A mobile arm support may assist the client in holding up his or her arm but most clients prefer to use as little equipment as possible. A scoop dish may be helpful but the universal cuff is necessary because the client will not have hand function. The electric wheelchair is not necessary for feeding but the client should be able to use a lightweight manual chair.

33. Answer: A

Suspended equipment such as swings are effective in treating vestibular disorders.

34. Answer: A

Scatter rugs are dangerous to everyone. They are often the cause of many home accidents, particularly to those with visual or mobility issues. Scatter rugs are often the cause of falls in the elderly.

35. Answer: D

Often older people lose their sight and do not want to learn Braille. The elderly usually prefer to adjust their environment with cues such as a rubber band on the orange juice but not on the milk.

36. Answer: B

Cross training means that several disciplines can provide for a patient's basic needs. For example, the psychologist can assist the client with using the bathroom, the occupational therapist can assist the client with ambulation.

37. Answer: A

Critical paths or pathways are predetermined treatment plans for routine treatments. For example, a rehabilitation program may have a critical path for a person with a total hip replacement that lays out what is to be reached at days 1, 3, and 5 of rehabilitation. Although critical paths may seem cookie cutter treatment plans, they are effective in typical patient progress and reduce documentation needs on the occupational therapist.

38. Answer: A

Discharge plans are most effective when begun at admission. This is true in both medical and psychiatric admissions and provides a focus for the treatment plan.

39. Answer: A

Use of a gentle touch and unhurried motions will reassure the patient.

40. Answer: B

Avoid twisting your body for all lifts.

41. Answer: D

Do not hose a wheelchair with water or let it air dry. Wipe it clean with a metal cleaner available in the car care section of department stores. Do not use a light oil on any part of the wheelchair as it will collect dirt. Use a molybdenum-based grease on the cross brace every 6 months. Educate your patients to follow the owner's manual.

42. Answer: A

Aspiration is life threatening and occurs when food passes through the larynx and into the lungs. Up to 60% of a nursing home population may need a swallowing program.

43. Answer: A

People with arthritis often have problems with bathing and these signs should not be confused with the dementia. B, C, and D have issues with ADLs in general, not just bathing.

44. Answer: B

All are signs of EPS except inability to sustain tongue movements. EPS includes increased movement in tongue both in and out of the mouth. In addition, EPS can include jaw biting, clenching, chewing, or mouth open.

45. Answer: B

Have client repeat information back by asking: "We have covered a lot of information today, can you summarize all the important information for me?" Always use the word medicine instead of pills or drugs. Avoid technical words altogether and never change the medication bottles. If the client is having a hard time with the bottles, encourage the client to ask the pharmacist to change the bottles for him or her.

46. Answer: B

Elderly that are cognitively impaired, such as dementia, do well in structure programs with activities, however, too many choices can be confusing. Validating feelings can greatly reduce anxiety. Names and pictures on doors help the resident find his or her room.

47. Answer: B

Wandering elderly are often confused as well. Bells on their shoes may act as an alarm but not likely. A safe environment inside and closed outside allows wandering without danger.

48. Answer: A

Closure activities is the last stage on the five-stage group. This includes closing on a positive note, asserting internal control, expressing pleasure, and leaving appropriately.

49. Answer: B

Mildred Ross describes this as a calming activity.

50. Answer: B

Although the KELS measures ADLs, it is a test developed to use once and predict ability to live independently. C and D are pediatric assessments. The Barthel can be used for functional outcome measures as well as patient evaluation.

SECTION FOUR

1. Answer: D

The infant's lower lip drops, the tongue moves forward, and the head turns when the rooting reflex is stimulated. This reflex can persist up to 7 months while the infant is asleep and is important to feeding. The grasp reflex is secondary to pressure on the palm of an infant. The galant reflex involves stroking the skin between the 12th rib and iliac crest. It persists in the newborn for 2 months. The primary righting reflex is elicited with pressure on the feet, ankles kneaded, or nape of neck tickled.

2. Answer: D

A member of good standing in AOTA has paid dues, followed the code of ethics, and met any other qualifications. A significant contribution to the field is awarded with honors but is not required to be in good standing.

3. Answer: B

Goal directed (level 4) actions use visual cues. Basic ADLs are performed, but nonvisual safety hazards are unrecognized. Attention span is about 1 hour. Level 5 uses trial and error, can recall several steps, and can complete basic ADLs. Level 6 is the highest level and represents no disability. Level 3 can perform manual actions with tactile cues. Attention span is about 30 minutes and needs repetition of steps.

4. Answer: B

A simple, familiar task with limited steps and visual cues is best. "Simon Says" is best for level 2. Budgeting and a model airplane are best for level 5.

5. Answer: A

Although all answers have merit, patient load requirements has the greatest impact on the number of staff required. OTRs who treat each patient 2 hours per day cannot treat as many patients as OTRs who treat each patient for 30 minutes per day.

6. Answer: D

AOTA membership is open to OTRs, COTAs, and OT students.

7. Answer: D

Occupational performance areas of Uniform Terminology include self-care, work, and play/leisure.

8. Answer: C

A classic sign of neglect is noted when half of the body is neglected in shaving, dressing, or washing. Motor apraxia would be a sequencing problem. Ideational apraxia would be noted if the patient were handed a shirt and the patient did not know what to do with it. Astereognosis is the inability to identify objects through touch alone.

9. Answer: C

MMT is invalid when a client does not have voluntary control of muscle function. A, B, and D would all benefit from ongoing assessment of muscle function.

10. Answer: B

The body surface is divided into areas of 9% or multiples of 9%.

11. Answer: D

Allowing the patient to control the AROM helps to control the level of pain.

12. Answer: A

The rotator cuff muscles include the "SIT" muscles: supraspinatus, infraspinatus, and teres minor. Subscapularis is an anterior cuff muscle. C and D are not cuff muscles.

13. Answer: A

Neurosis appears as a symptom. Reality testing is intact. Anxiety, somatoform, dissociative, sexual, and dysthymic disorders are examples. Psychosis is not reality bound. Mental disorder is distress or disability from behavioral, biological, or psychological cause. Dysphoria is an unpleasant mood.

14. Answer: B

Only NBCOT administers the OTR exam.

15. Answer: D

Any person can make a referral to an occupational therapist; however, third party insurance providers often require a physician's order for reimbursement of services.

16. Answer: D

The triceps are innervated by C7 and C8. Deltoid, biceps, and serratus anterior are innervated at C5 or above.

17. Answer: A

Guillain-Barré is a lower motor neuron disease. B, C, and D are not true.

18. Answer: D

Motor weakness, paralysis, sensory loss, and compromised respiratory system are all symptoms of Guillain-Barré.

19. Answer: C

The best choice for the first day is setting up a device to call the nurse.

20. Answer: C

Transference is a psychoanalytic term used to describe projected thoughts or feelings onto the therapist who represents someone from the past. Consensual validation is when group members check their perceptions with other group members. Therapist transparency is when the therapist reveals more about him- or herself to confirm or disconfirm the patient's perception. Counter transference refers to the therapist's projection onto the patient.

21. Answer: D

Although all the activities provide either some tactile input or some kinesthetic awareness, rolling on the wall provides both.

22. Answer: A

The executive director of AOTA is a full-time employee of the association. Policies of AOTA are approved by the representative assembly (RA). The ethics committee or the RA does not elect the executive director.

23. Answer: C

This situation is common in practice. The OTR should call the doctor and initiate a professional conversation about the assessment and suggested treatment.

24. Answer: C

Autonomic dysreflexia includes symptoms of increased perspiration, flushing, and headache.

25. Answer: A

Autonomic dysreflexia is an immediate medical emergency. Keep the patient upright and get medical assistance immediately. Do check the leg bag tubing for obstruction but do not continue treatment.

26. Answer: C

Liver or kidney disease may affect the patient's interest in food, diet requirements, or digestion, but does not affect swallowing.

27. Answer: A

B, C, and D can cause a coma in a person with Alzheimer's disease. A head injury from a fall may appear to be a seizure. The MI is less likely to be the cause of the coma unless it resulted in anoxia.

28. Answer: D

Over-the-counter medicines can also cause adverse drug reactions, especially when mixed with prescriptions. The longer an individual is on a medication the greater the likelihood of drug reactions. Drugs are a major cause of dizziness in persons over age 60.

29. Answer: C

Increased ambulation does improve unsteadiness but appropriate footwear that provides support must be worn. A, B, and D provide additional alternatives to restraints.

30. Answer: A

Mildred Ross describes this as an alerting activity.

31. Answer: B

This approach is evidence of a power struggle and is often perceived as threatening by the patient who can easily become defensive. A, C, and D are all behavioral techniques aimed at increasing positive reinforcement to increase desired behaviors.

32. Answer: A

Newborns to youth have the highest frequency of epilepsy. Numbers decrease in the 11 to 69 age range and then increase again at 70 due to increased health problems and medications.

33. Answer: A

Hypotonic muscles are low tone that leads to lack of support of joints. Spastic muscles are hypertonic. B, C, and D are all complications of spasticity.

34. Answer: C

The function of the cerebellum is the execution of smooth, coordinated, and properly timed movement. Ataxic gait is an incoordinated gait. Hypotonia is a decrease in muscle tone. Dysmetria is the inability to direct movement and is characterized by reaching past objects. Dysdiadochokinesia is the inability for rapid, repeated, alternating movements. Clinical signs of parietal lobe damage include sensory disorders, apraxia, and perceptual problems. Clinical signs of premotor cortex damage include motor apraxia and difficulty with tasks that require sensory guidance. Clinical signs of basal ganglia damage include akinesia, bradykinesia, dystonia, and perseveration.

35. Answer: B

Eclecticism refers to the selection and organized blending of compatible features from a variety of sources. Object relations is a blending of humanistic-existential, Freudian, and Jungian theories. A and C are specific frames of reference that have been researched for measurable outcomes. D is not a frame of reference but refers to Fidler's group model.

36. Answer: C

Vestibular treatment with swings or suspended equipment is most effective although the fixed monkey bars may be able to provide some movement. A and D provide no movement and therefore no treatment, however, are likely to be preferred by a child with vestibular problems.

37. Answer: D

Almost all adults experience some sensation with over half experiencing pain. Phantom pain does disturb body image but may aid in rehabilitation in that the patient continues to have body perception during training. Phantom pain exists because the neurological scheme continues after loss of the actual limb.

38. Answer: D

The clock drawing task is a non-standardized but effective tool to evaluate perceptual problems often seen in those people with CVAs and left-sided weakness. The task is perceptual, not cognitive, and does not evaluate the ability to tell time.

39. Answer: C

The MAP is a preschool screening test designed to assess developmental delays in preacademic skills. The MAI-ST identifies movement patterns in infants 2 to 18 months. The EDPA measures changes in hand functioning. The Peabody assesses fine and gross motor skills in children up to age 7 years.

40. Answer: A

This activity could estimate cognitive functioning and increase a person's self-knowledge. B is sensory integrative in its approach. C is part of the habituation subsystem in the model of human occupation, and D is part of object relations theory.

41. Answer: D

Although serious complications can be associated with spasticity, there are some important benefits also associated. Spasticity aids in the prevention of osteoporosis due to the pressure exerted on the bone by the muscle. Calcium loss from the bone is decreased. Muscle atrophy is prevented due to the contracted state of the muscle. Prevention of DVT is achieved by a decreased probability of blood pooling in the lower extremities when spasticity is present.

42. Answer: A

Executive function includes the ability to organize and carry out a task. This includes making decisions, sequencing, problem solving, and judgment. B, C, and D are tested in perceptual evaluations.

43. Answer: B

Gradation is adapting an activity higher or lower to provide adequate challenge but guarantee success in the patient. All other answers are false.

44. Answer: A

Good listening skills include all of the answers except the therapist should lean slightly forward toward the client. Facing the client, maintaining eye contact, and appearing relaxed and open tells the client "I'm here for you."

45. Answer: A

Level I, no response, and level II, generalized response, are appropriate for sensory stimulation. Level III, localized response, may further benefit but they can begin to handle other activities.

46. Answer: D

Level IV, confused agitated, is a heightened state of activity with agitation. Sensory stimulation would not be appropriate for this client as it would likely confuse the client more.

47. Answer: C

Level VI is the confused but appropriate level where clients benefit from repetition and practice in a safe environment. The levels before VI are confused, inappropriate, or agitated and tasks may not be practiced successfully. Level VII is community based, practice is in the community.

48. Answer: A

Cognitive rehabilitation is most heavy in levels V and VI with complex tasks managed at level VII. Level VIII would have mastered the skills.

49. Answer: B

Leaving or confronting a person with delusions isolates the person. Delusions are unreal beliefs that cannot be cleared with facts. Until the person's thoughts clear with medication, the best approach is to validate the person's feelings without feeding into the delusion.

50. Answer: B

A, C, and D require too much attention for this patient to successfully complete. The tie-dyed t-shirt is a success-oriented project because even if mistakes are made because the client is distracted, the shirt will usually come out well.

SECTION FIVE

1. Answer: D

Industrial prevention programs and education in chronic pain programs are essential roles in occupational therapy. A, B, and C are components of prevention and retraining education.

2. Answer: D

Anxiety must be dealt with first to address immediate physical limitations and long-term lifestyle changes. A, B, and C are important treatment components but are secondary to reducing anxiety.

3. Answer: C

The BTE is commonly used for evaluation and treatment in a work rehabilitation program. Although the BTE might be used for cardiac rehabilitation, it is unlikely to be used for motor learning after a CVA or for sensory integration programs.

4. Answer: A

Spontaneous play is an essential component of a child's work.

5. Answer: B

The OTR must keep in mind the target audience when developing presentations. This audience would benefit from learning about the problems adults with mental illness face and how OT can address the weaknesses.

6. Answer: B

Medicare is for those age 65 and over. Medicaid is a state health program for the poor. SSI/SSD is income for people over age 65 or people with disabilities. Welfare and section 8 are state income programs for the poor.

7. Answer: D

Although documentation can help a health care professional in case there is an ethical claim, the purpose of documentation is to protect the consumer. Research, communication, and serial records are all benefits of proper documentation.

8. Answer: A

Thought insertion is a delusion where the patient believes that thoughts are being implanted by an outside force. Delusions of reference is the belief that behavior of others refers to oneself. Hypervigilance is continuous scanning of the environment for self-protection. Magical thinking is believing one has magical powers to cause something to happen.

9. Answer: D

The occupational therapist should consider using empathy to minimize tensions because the patient is delusional. This response, unlike the others, will convey understanding and assist in establishing rapport. A, B, and C will likely increase the patient's defenses.

10. Answer: D

Focus groups, surveys, demographics, questionnaires, key informants, and literature reviews are all excellent sources of data for a needs assessment. Etiology information is not helpful unless it directly relates to a high environmental incidence in your area. Needs assessments focus on the need for services not the cause of diseases.

11. Answer: A

All of the answers are important to the treatment of RSD, however, edema should be the therapist's first concern.

12. Answer: B

The wrist extensors are innervated by the radial nerve. Thumb and little finger opposition can be a median nerve test. Gross grasp is not a specific test. Pinching the thumb and index finger can be an ulnar nerve test. More detailed evaluation is needed to specifically identify median/ulnar problems.

13. Answer: D

Dependency needs in the early phase of adjustment to a chronic disease can be seen in chronic pain, multiple sclerosis, arthritis, and other long-term diseases.

14. Answer: D

Swan neck can be caused by other factors but the classic position is PIP hyperextension and DIP flexion. MCP subluxation is articular instability secondary to capsular weakness and muscle imbalance. DIP hyperextension and PIP flexion is boutonniere deformity. MCP ulnarly deviated is generally associated with weak collateral ligaments.

15. Answer: C

The symptoms most closely resemble a manic episode of bipolar disorder.

16. Answer: B

The patient genuinely believes that he is a famous person who has achieved great accomplishment. An unreal belief is a delusion. Hallucinations are perceptual, not cognitive. There is no suggestion of paranoid thinking. Malingering is an intentional act to deceive and is not considered a mental disorder.

17. Answer: D

The patient must be able to modify his own behavior to the environment to accomplish the other goals mentioned. A, B, and C are relevant after poor self-control is stabilized first.

18. Answer: A

A tile box project would provide structure and repetition to sustain attention and attain mastery. The puzzle and budgeting are too lengthy and unstructured for the initial treatment sessions. Wood carving should be avoided due to the sharp utensils until the patient is stabilized.

19. Answer: D

One splint alone will not be sufficient; all are required.

20. Answer: B

Due to the stretch of the extensors over more than one joint, the length of the muscle would not allow full flexion to occur.

21. Answer: C

Playing dog involves extended arms and head movement. Spinning on a scooter board is a vestibular activity. The balance beam activity may be too advanced for this child. Marbles are a fine motor activity.

22. Answer: C

The NBCOT exam can be taken only after all classwork and fieldwork are completed. State licensure requires applicants to have completed the NBCOT process.

23. Answer: C

Measurable, observable, realistic, explicit.

24. Answer: A

The philosophy and mission statement are the foundation for the existing programs as well as the new program. Goals, objectives, patient services, and documentation are developed only after the philosophy and mission statement are reviewed.

25. Answer: C

Scoliosis is often noted in young females. Routine testing in schools throughout the country screens for this lateral curvature of the spine.

26. Answer: B

The SIPT requires pediatric experience, specific training, and knowledge of statistics and measurement. Three courses are offered by Sensory Integration International. The Sensory Rating Scale is for ages 0 to 3 years and takes 20 minutes to give. The Sensory Assessment is for ages 5 to 18 years and is standardized. The KSHQ is a questionnaire given to parents about their child's behavior.

27. Answer: C

This side effect makes sense if you think about the two diseases: Parkinson's and schizophrenia. People with Parkinson's have decreased level of dopamine and people with schizophrenia have too much dopamine. As the medication increases to improve movement, psychotic features may present.

28. Answer: A

Bending over is a concern for all the diagnoses listed, but holding their breath while bending over is of particular danger for cardiac patients as the two combined adds additional stress on the heart.

29. Answer: C

According to data collected in 1996, 80% of all people with epilepsy can be successfully treated. Although the disease is not cured, medication can reduce seizure activity modifying the disease process to reduce further damage to the CNS.

30. Answer: A

Central cord syndrome occurring in the cervical region results in sacral sensory sparing and greater weakness in the UE than the LE. B is Brown-Séquard syndrome. C is anterior cord syndrome. D is cauda equina syndrome.

31. Answer: C

The biomechanical factor shows that approximately 50% of the body weight is supported by the concept of buoyancy.

32. Answer: D

The MVPT provides a quick assessment of visual perceptual abilities without requiring the child to have motor skills. Since the child has cerebral palsy, motor skills may be a problem. Her age of 7 is within the age range of all the assessments.

33. Answer: D

When writing legislative letters, include all of the items, as well as address the letter correctly, keep comments to the point, and be respectful.

34. Answer: C

All of the items are false except C. It is important that the occupational therapist be aware of MRSA because the therapist is at risk of becoming infected or passing the infection on to others. Follow hospital guidelines for gowning, wearing gloves, and wearing eye protection.

35. Answer: D

The Fugl-Meyer Scale is a measure of motor recovery after stroke. All the other assessments include independent living skills subtests.

36. Answer: D

Pull out a paper towel so that it will be ready to dry your clean hands without touching the dispenser. Turn on the water and wet hands before adding soap. Rub hands and wrists vigorously for at least 15 seconds. Wash around rings, do not remove. Rinse well and dry hands. Use paper towel to turn off water. Do not touch wastebasket.

37. Answer: B

A gallon of milk weighs over 8 lbs (128 oz/16 oz per pound = 8 lbs plus the container weight). All the other items weigh about 2 lbs.

38. Answer: B

TTWB does not allow any weight but allows the toe to be used for balance. WBAT allows weight to be applied until pain. FWB has no restrictions.

39. Answer: C

Rotter called this general concept locus of control. Internal locus of control is when a personal feels personally responsible for life events rather than life events being controlled by outside influences. External locus of control refers to a belief that outside forces are causing events to happen. Competence is efficacy in meeting environmental demands.

40. Answer: A

Ability is a general trait referring to genetic influences and learning during one's life. Autonomy is shown by one's ability to make choices and have control over one's environment. Order refers to a desired, symptom-free state of being.

41. Answer: D

Allen's theory is suited for persons with physical and cognitive deficits who can benefit by learning how to compensate for his or her decreased abilities. A refers to Mosey's frame of role acquisition. B refers to a developmental frame such as Llorens'. C refers to the model of human occupation.

42. Answer: A

NSAIDs are inexpensive over-the-counter medications such as aspirin or ibuprofen. These are considered the frontline approach to the management of arthritis. NSAIDs are not disease modifying but do treat the symptoms.

43. Answer: B

The client is on a DMARD such as oral gold compound (Ridaura/auranofin) which attempts to halt the progression of arthritic changes. Gold has many side effects including skin rash, diarrhea, and irritation of the oral mucosa.

44. Answer: D

The client may have difficulty holding on to any longhandled piece of equipment. The bar stool may be a good idea, but since the client is living in her own home and has no cognitive problems, the best approach is for her to try out different pieces of equipment and then choose what she thinks will be most helpful.

45. Answer: D

Intentional tremor is a tremor on movement, usually seen in multiple sclerosis. The tremor associated with Parkinson's disease is a resting tremor or pill rolling movement. A, B, and C are characteristics of the disease.

46. Answer: A

A new OTR can supervise all levels of OT personnel except a Level II fieldwork student. The new graduate's supervision is not required but highly recommended.

47. Answer: B

A new graduate COTA must be supervised at the site with daily direct contact. Intermediate or advanced COTAs can have routine or general supervision.

48. Answer: A

Ayers believed that adaptive responses could be achieved when sensation is organized and situations provide a "just right" challenge with built-in success. B refers to Gilfoyle and Grady's frame of spatiotemporal adaptation which emphasizes the role of movement in one's environment. C refers to Reilly's occupational behavior which emphasizes humans' innate need to master their environment through play and work. D refers to Mosey's role acquisition where humans' desire for mastery leads to successful adaptation in a variety of roles including ADL, work, and play.

49. Answer: B

A defines impairment, C defines handicap, and D defines occupational performance dysfunction.

50. Answer: B

PAMs can be used by OT personnel when used in adjunct to or in preparation of purposeful activity. Simply using PAMs to reduce pain without OT treatment would not be part of occupational therapy.

SECTION SIX

1. Answer: B

Pressure garments and splinting are an integral part of the program to prevent scarring. PT and OT would work together to range the involved areas, however, only pressure garments prevent scarring. Nursing and family also play an important role.

2. Answer: A

Poor motor planning and sequencing problems indicate motor apraxia. Finding the soap is an example of a figure ground problem. Frustration could be a sign of many different problems. Understanding the directions is a receptive aphasia problem.

3. Answer: C

Decreased muscle tone, weak cocontraction, and decreased ability to resist gravity are all signs of hypotonicity. Hyperactive tendon reflexes are noted in spastic hypertonicity, the opposite condition.

4. Answer: B

Clients with head injuries often require a structured pre work hardening program that emphasizes work and social skills. At this time the client is ready for treatment but not ready for a work hardening program. The client does need to work in a group to develop skills, however, does not need inpatient hospital services. An inpatient program requires continuing medical instability.

5. Answer: A

Group norms are also known as rules of conduct. Group roles refers to the part one plays in a group. Subgrouping refers to speaking with certain members and excluding others. Task roles refers to the role taken by members to address tasks at hand.

6. Answer: C

Vestibular stimulation has been correlated with increased verbalization, responsiveness, and muscle tone. Self-care may benefit if the child is directed to perform self-care activities. Behavioral modification techniques are helpful to address ADLs.

7. Answer: C

Informal evaluation of a client's AROM does provide the OTR with initial information regarding muscle strength. The client must have a fair grade in order to achieve AROM against gravity. The therapist must provide resistance to assess a good grade, palpate to assess the end feel, or use PROM to establish joint play.

8. Answer: C

Slow rocking will result in dampening the vestibuloproprioceptors and decreasing tone throughout the body. Slow rolling and a quiet environment will also decrease tone.

9. Answer: D

The suture joint is a fibrous joint such as a skull suture. Hinge, saddle, and ball and socket all have characteristics of diarthrodial or synovial joints such as synovium, joint space, synovial fluid, or capsules.

10. Answer: C

Concentric is muscle shortening, isometric is no change in muscle length, and isotonic is muscle shortening.

11. Answer: C

Making eye contact, smiling, and nodding are all social reinforcers. Therapeutic self-disclosure is a skill an occupational therapist uses to support the client gaining a new awareness about him- or herself.

12. Answer: D

Too much vestibular input can cause emotional responses.

13. Answer: B

Process is the act of recognizing, examining, and understanding the nature of interpersonal relationships. Therapeutic dynamics refers to the forces within a group. Explicit words refer to the content. Therapeutic interventions refers to the technique.

14. Answer: A

The problem-oriented medical record is a type of documentation system.

15. Answer: D

Isometric exercises will reduce stress on the joint structure while exercising the soft tissue.

16. Answer: B

During supination, the proximal end of the radius spins within the radial notch. The distal end slides over the ulnar head.

17. Answer: D

Diagnosis related groups are categories that suggest the acceptable length of stay in the hospital for each diagnosis.

18. Answer: C

Repetition will help the client learn parts of the prosthetic device, enhance body scheme adjustment, allow gradation, allow for decrease of therapist cues, and will allow the client to desensitize himself to the emotional aspects of amputation. Strengthening and stump care are important, but only after adjustment issues have been addressed.

19. Answer: B

Bending while sitting and crossing legs or ankles can all lead to dislocating the hip joint. Walking is safe and healthy as long as the weather is good.

20. Answer: D

Egocentric-cooperative is the correct term. At this stage members select and implement a long-term task. At the parallel level, individuals will work side by side. At the cooperative level the therapist is an advisor. Members can satisfy each other's social and emotional needs. Project level groups emphasize a task accomplishment with some interaction. Group development moves from parallel, project, egocentric-cooperative, cooperative, and finally to mature.

21. Answer: B

Occupational therapists can refer patients to any appropriate health care professional.

22. Answer: C

There are no clear clinical signs to detect hypertension predictably. Blood pressure must be monitored. Many people exhibit shortness of breath (SOB) for a variety of reasons. SOB may not be an indicator of high blood pressure. Headaches can occur with hypertension but also for many other reasons. Dizziness can occur with both hypertension and hypotension, as well as for other reasons.

23. Answer: B

If the arches of the hand are not maintained, deformity of the hand could result. Fit is enhanced with proper strap placement to avoid skin breakdown from rubbing.

24. Answer: A

The volitional system serves at the top of the hierarchy and energizes other subsystems to achieve goals. The three components include personal causation, values, and interests. Habituation components include roles and habits. Organization of daily activities is the main function. Performance includes skills needed to perform purposeful activities: perceptual motor, process, communication, and interactive skills. Environment is not a subsystem.

25. Answer: D

The Mini Mental Status is an excellent screening tool to track a patient's cognitive state over time. Although a formal evaluation of cognitive impairment may be done as a psychological test, the Mini Mental Status exam includes areas of orientation, registration, calculation, recall, language, and construction. The ACL is a cognitive test but does not address the above areas. The BaFPE includes cognitive, affective, and psychomotor. The KELS is best suited for readiness for discharge in the ADL area.

26. Answer: A

PAMs are not considered part of entry-level practice but require specialized learning. An OTR can delegate the use of PAMs to a COTA with training but as with all media, shall comply with all supervision requirements to ensure competency. OT personnel can use PAMs even if physical therapists are available or when reimbursement is not available as long as the personnel comply with state licensure laws.

27. Answer: B

The administration of Levodopa often dramatically improves symptoms, especially rigidity and bradykinesia. It remains the most common drug for the treatment of Parkinson's disease. Valium is an anti-anxiety medication. NSAIDs are anti-inflammatory and heparin is an anti-coagulant.

28. Answer: B

Although A, C, and D might provide support, the dynamic extension splint provides the best treatment for wrist drop.

29. Answer: D

A full visual field is represented by 180° of vision without moving the eyes. A and B are structures in the eye. Visual acuity is the sharpness of vision.

30. Answer: C

The first step is to attain strengths and weaknesses in an initial screening and assessment followed by answer A. D is part of treatment planning.

31. Answer: A

Puréed food has a bland taste which added to all the other factors may make it difficult to swallow. B, C, and D are all true.

32. Answer: B

Depression is likely the cause. All the other diagnoses would have additional signs.

33. Answer: D

Not to be used due to high sodium. The therapist should watch for signs of edema or congestive heart failure if the patient states he or she has been taking this medication and inform the client to stop taking the medicine until consulting with the physician.

34. Answer: B

Childhood includes 6 to 12 years, young adulthood is 20 to 35 years, and middle adulthood is 35 to 50 years.

35. Answer: C

In avoidant coping, attention is focused away from the stressful source. Cognitive strategies include reasoning, appraising, and reflection. Behavioral strategies include taking action to the source of the stress. Problem-focused coping includes doing something constructive to work out the problem.

36. Answer: D

Persons with impairments in executive functioning can verbally discuss their behavior but have difficulty doing or initiating action.

37. Answer: C

The right-sided weakness indicates CVA.

38. Answer: C

A, B, and D are valuable but the client leads the therapy, especially true in home care.

39. Answer: D

This client did not have another stroke as evidenced by no decrease in motoric abilities. She likely had digitalis toxicity. The client's decrease in mobility after the stroke influenced her metabolism and excretion of the digitalis, so the same dose that was effective before the stroke is now toxic.

40. Answer: A

All the acts have influences on the education of children in the United States.

41. Answer: A

Vertical righting reactions include body righting. They are not present at birth but develop with interaction with the environment. Turning the head is part of rotational righting reactions.

42. Answer: C

Flexor withdrawal, crossed extension, and Bauer's are tested with touch pressure to the foot.

43. Answer: A

The olfactory system is a primitive, chemically based sensory system that signals the CNS about smells.

44. Answer: B

Emphasis is placed on the process of the group, not the actual end product. All other statements reflect Fidler's task group model researched at the New York Psychiatric Institute in 1965.

45. Answer: A

The other three official AOTA papers are important policies that influence education and practice of occupational therapy.

46. Answer: D

Fidler observed in her research at the New York Psychiatric Institute how patients with schizophrenia felt threatened by the act of "doing." This doing in a task group actually demonstrated their skills and functioning level. A, B, and C are not performance based.

47. Answer: B

OT practitioners are only OTRs and COTAs who are certified to practice. OT aides or technicians require intense, close supervision by the OTR and/or COTA.

48. Answer: D

In addition, the paper also describes the roles of faculty, program director, researcher, and scholar.

49. Answer: C

This is the definition used in Uniform Terminology. Coping skills are defined as identifying and managing stress. Self-expression is the use of various styles and skills to express thoughts, feelings, and needs. Values are identified ideas and beliefs considered personally important.

50. Answer: D

Immediacy is effectively used to discuss issues that develop between the client and the occupational therapist. An important part of immediacy is inviting the client to examine the relationship.

SECTION SEVEN

1. Answer: C

This is the hallmark sign for delirium versus dementia. Dementia is a syndrome which includes cognitive impairments without impairment in consciousness.

2. Answer: B

A significant issue for people with substance dependency is organizing a social network that is supportive. Since substance abuse often becomes the primary focus of activity, a significant OT goal is time management and the restructuring of social activities to prevent slippage. A and D can also be helpful.

3. Answer: A

Infancy is considered from 0 to 18 months and ends when the child is able to speak. Creeping occurs at about 40 weeks. Climbing stairs occurs around 2 years. Bowel control occurs around 3 years.

4. Answer: B

AOTF's primary goal is the development of research in occupational therapy. In addition, AOTF provides scholarships, fundraising, and houses the occupational therapy library.

5. Answer: D

The movable arm is parallel to the humerus midline. B and C are not involved.

6. Answer: C

People with amputation spend more energy during ADL than people without amputations. Adaptive equipment might help, however, energy conservation is first. Supervising others and cognitive retraining are only appropriate if there are deficiencies in these areas.

7. Answer: B

There would be loss of AROM. Supraspinatus assists with shoulder abduction. Other muscles would compensate to allow some movement. PROM is usually normal in rotator cuff injuries.

8. Answer: C

Panic attacks have a sudden onset that can reach a peak within 10 minutes. Other signs include trembling, sensation of shortness of breath, feeling of choking, chest pain, nausea, derealization, fear of dying, paralysis, and chills. Generalized anxiety is chronic and persistent. It is always possible that the patient might be having a heart attack and should be checked. Stress is a generalized term.

9. Answer: D

Safety of the patient is always the first priority. While other responses are relevant, the initial responsibility is to secure the patient.

10. Answer: C

Upper trapezius and levator scapula are the primary movers for scapula elevation. Rhomboids assist when trapezius is weak. Sternocleidomastoid flexes the neck. Pectoralis minor can act as a downward rotator of the scapula.

11. Answer: B

The certification exam for the COTA is completely different from the exam for the OTR.

12. Answer: B

Energy conservation and work simplification are the priorities after safety and might lead to adaptive equipment. Although balance enhancement exercises would be helpful, the fatigue must be addressed first. A home health aide might be helpful but would reduce the client's sense of independence and increase the feeling of loss of self-control.

13. Answer: D

Neck righting is an upper brainstem induced reflex indicating a refined postural adjustment. Flexor withdrawal, extensor thrust, and positive supporting reaction are all spinal reflexes.

14. Answer: C

Management by objective is a common approach to managing occupational therapy departments and other health care programs.

15. Answer: B

Medicare does not assign the cost of equipment; however, it is expected that the cost will be comparable to local costs for that item. Durable medical equipment paid for under Medicare must withstand repeated use, be used for medical purposes, and be useless in absence of illness or injury.

16. Answer: A

There is no significant increase in paranoid ideas in the following cultural groups: African-Americans, Caucasians, or Native Americans. Recent immigrants have a higher rate of developing delusional disorder due to the uncertainty of their new environment. Immigrants must adjust to new people with different mannerisms, responses, and language.

17. Answer: A

Although other areas of intervention would be valuable, working on integration of primitive reflexes will enhance overall development. Visual tracking and eye-hand coordination can be addressed after the reflexes. Small pegs are too difficult and dangerous for any 1-year-old.

18. Answer: B

PNF is a classic movement treatment approach developed in the late 1940s. PNF uses the theory of diagonal or spinal movement as essential for motor control and the basis for normal movement. Rood uses a developmental sequence as a prerequisite for recovery. Icing and brush are Rood techniques. Brunnstrom focuses on synergy status and the stages of recovery. Bobath places emphasis on reflex inhibiting postures (RIP) and key point of control.

19. Answer: B

The directive group is designed for patients with minimal functioning who are often excluded from traditional group treatment. A, C, and D are true of a directive group.

20. Answer: B

The president of AOTA is elected by the membership. The president is a volunteer position unlike the executive director of AOTA.

21. Answer: C

The hip is a ball and socket joint that allows flexion/extension, rotation, and abduction/adduction.

22. Answer: A

Delirium is a syndrome, not a disease. Delirium has many causes that result in a pattern of symptoms. These symptoms include impairment in consciousness and cognitive deficits. Neurological signs include tremor, nystagmus, incoordination, and urinary incontinence.

23. Answer: D

Expressive arts such as art, dance, movement, and writing are excellent resources to increase a patient's understanding of her dynamics and related feelings. A, B, and C are task-oriented modalities.

24. Answer: A

Collateral ligaments are designed to be taught in flexion to check the movement of the digits at the joint. They act as a stability function.

25. Answer: B

The muscles of the hand form two masses in the palm. These are the thenar at the base of the thumb and the hypothenar eminence at the base of the little finger.

26. Answer: C

Although A, B, and D are relevant in the initial treatment stage, the OTR should shift focus to the caregiver at discharge. Since this is a progressive disorder, the caregivers should be prepared for emerging deficits. The OTR can learn from the caregiver about the patient's individual needs to customize the discharge plan.

27. Answer: D

Skin breakdown is common, especially for people with LEAK amputation. Often skin breakdown is caused by poor socket fit or wrinkles in the stump sock. Adaptive equipment and donning training are important after the priority of skin care. Gait training will likely be addressed by physical therapy with OT assisting in safety issues.

28. Answer: A

Uniform Terminology is an official document of AOTA and defines the practice of occupational therapy. It includes occupational performance areas and occupational performance components. Uniform Terminology is used in developing the examination questions for the OTR registration exam. If you have gotten this far in your studies and are not familiar with Uniform Terminology, we suggest you quickly get a copy for review (see Chapter One for further information).

29. Answer: A

Carpal tunnel syndrome involves the median nerve.

30. Answer: C

A soft end feel is compression of tissue and feels soft, not firm, abrupt, or capsular. A and B are not pathological; D is an abnormal condition.

31. Answer: D

Dementia from Alzheimer's, vascular disease, and AIDS is not reversible. Depression in the elderly is often confused with dementia because the patient presents with confusion and memory impairment. Also known as pseudo dementia, this depression is most likely treatable and reversible.

32. Answer: B

All OTR and COTA educational programs must maintain accreditation with AOTA. Programs without accreditation cannot have their graduates sit for the registration exam. Without taking the exam, graduates are unable to practice occupational therapy.

33. Answer: C

Documentation is covered by the code of ethics under communication that contains false, fraudulent, deceptive, or unfair statements (AOTA, 1994).

34. Answer: C

The first action is to speak to the therapist who made the comment. Although it may be uncomfortable, as an occupational therapist it is your duty to stop an unethical practice. If the therapist continues with the plan to bill ahead, speak to a supervisor. If the supervisor does not stop the practice, report the information to the standards and ethics committee (SEC) of AOTA. The SEC will provide you with information and support on how to handle the problem. Ethical problems are always difficult to address, but as an OTR you have a high standard to protect our consumers.

35. Answer: D

The biomechanical frame of reference (FOR) looks at forces affecting function. Orthopedic conditions use MMT, goniometry, and strength training to improve function. Kinematics is inherent in this intervention, therefore, the biomechanical FOR is appropriate. Sensory motor FOR is generally employed when CNS damage has occurred. Cognitive and developmental FOR are not appropriate for orthopedic conditions as the therapist can assume that no cognitive or development issues are present as primary issues in treatment.

36. Answer: D

Parachute games provide noncompetitive sensorimotor activity. Researchers theorize that perceptual, posture, body image, and motor planning deficits found in patients with schizophrenia are the result of poor sensory integration. Tennis and basketball are competitive. Walking is unstructured and not as stimulating as parachute games.

37. Answer: C

The right CVA with left involved extremities would have a hemianopsia of the left nasal side of the right eye and the left temporal side of the left eye.

38. Answer: C

Spasticity is a condition of hypertonia. Athetoid is associated with hypotonia. The client would have full PROM but decreased coordination. Flaccid muscles are seen in extreme hypotonia. Ataxia is also within the hypotonic range with decreased coordination and controlled movement.

39. Answer: D

   While other goals can be integrated, visual memory is primary to the game.

40. Answer: C

   Social smiling occurs between 4 to 8 weeks. Infant smiles are endogenous and apparent in blind infants as well as sighted infants. Visual fixation occurs between 2 to 4 weeks. Spontaneous social smiling is evident at 16 weeks.

41. Answer: D

   Medicare will pay for a trapeze if used by someone confined to bed and needed for mobility. Medicare will pay for a splint if used to increase or restore function. Medicare will pay for a bedside commode if used by someone confined to a room. Medicare will not pay for grab bars because these are considered self-help items.

42. Answer: D

   The disturbance cannot be due to direct physiological effects of a substance. Social dysfunction, delusions, and disorganized speech are among the symptoms needed to diagnosis someone with schizophrenia. Other symptoms include hallucinations, disorganized speech, negative symptoms, occupational dysfunction, and grossly disorganized or catatonic behavior. Negative symptoms include flat affect, alogia, and avolition.

43. Answer: C

   The WFOT is composed of OTs around the world. Members do not have to be AOTA registered, however, therapists can pay their WFOT dues when they pay their AOTA dues.

44. Answer: A

   Acceptance facilitation is an important role for occupational therapy. The OTR can do this in conjunction with the prosthesis training. Anger can be addressed in acceptance. Independence instead of dependency is the goal of OT. Adaptive equipment will help in all areas of acceptance but must be appropriately timed.

45. Answer: C

   Piaget defines egocentrism as behavior typical of 2- to 7-year-olds in the stage of preoperational thought. Children in this stage feel they are the center of the universe, have a limited point of view, and are not capable of empathizing with others. A child at this stage is not being negativistic. Symbolization is the ability of an infant to create an image of an object. Imminent justice is the belief that punishment for wrong doing is inevitable.

46. Answer: B

   Because the child is not doing anything wrong, educating the parent is the most supportive. Although redirecting the child may stop the behavior, the best response is parent education.

47. Answer: B

   Hearing voices is the most common hallucination in schizophrenia with visual as second most common. Visual hallucinations alone are more common with people in detoxification programs for drugs and alcohol. Tactile and olfactory hallucinations are less common.

48. Answer: A

The wallet includes the most steps in reasoning, decision making, problem solving, and performance. A discussion group is open ended and unstructured. A movement or dance group usually includes aspects of sensorimotor or projective arts. Drawing a person is typical of the psychoanalytic frame of reference.

49. Answer: A

Medicare requires a durable medical equipment prescription from a physician to include the diagnosis, prognosis, reason for need, and estimation for the length of need. The cost does not need to be included in the order.

50. Answer: B

Common symptoms of depression are decreased pleasure or interest in activities, fatigue, and decreased energy. Reality orientation is awareness of person, place, and time. There is no indication of this problem. Responsibility and problem solving cannot be judged due to limited data. Further assessment is needed.

SECTION EIGHT

1. Answer: C

Physical therapy is out of the expertise of both the facility staff and the OTR. A, B, and D are all roles of the consulting OTR.

2. Answer: A

Universal precautions should be applied to blood and other fluids containing blood. Feces, urine, sweat, and tears have extremely low to nonexistent rates of HIV infection unless they include blood. Universal precautions include gloves, gowns, face guards, and cleaning with bleach and water. The therapist may choose to wear gloves when treating all patients to reduce spreading germs to the patient. Washing hands before and after all treatment is general good practice.

3. Answer: C

Taking a long shower before applying make-up may be too exhausting. Energy conservation is the priority for this teenager. A, B, and D will all help conserve energy.

4. Answer: D

At approximately 12 to 18 months, children can show various emotions such as distress, anger, fear, sadness, and shame. At 3 to 4 years they can feel guilt. Sitting alone, creeping, and saying one word are all developmentally appropriate landmarks for 40 weeks.

5. Answer: A

Joint Commission on Accreditation of Healthcare Organizations.

6. Answer: D

Increased heart rate, dilated pupils, and increased salivary secretions are all sympathetic.

7. Answer: A

People with AIDS are prone to Kaposi's sarcoma, pneumocystic carinii pneumonia, and toxoplasmosis. Amyotrophic lateral sclerosis is a neurological disorder with onset between 40 to 70 years old.

8. Answer: D

Ergonomics is the science of workplace design.

9. Answer: D

A single switch is for a person with only gross hand movements. Keyboards and joysticks require finger gross motor or some fine motor.

10. Answer: D

State laws vary, however, the OTR is usually mandated to report the incident to the appropriate authority. Most states have a department of family services, which is responsible for investigating suspected abusive situations. If you are not sure who to call, ask your local police department for the child protection agency phone number.

11. Answer: A

Decision making is difficult for a person with COPD only if the blood gases are off. Eating, speaking, and exercising are always difficult if not impossible.

12. Answer: D

140/90 is normal for someone under 40 years old. 160/90 is considered normal if the person is over age 40.

13. Answer: B

A child's awareness of space and direction helps him or her read left to right and place words on paper. Sorting and drawing represents body image which begins during infancy. Picking objects out is an example of figure ground.

14. Answer: B

Speak at a normal speed, tone, and volume. Keep hands away from your face, get the person's attention before starting, and talk face to face.

15. Answer: B

Body image is a major aspect of OT treatment for people with eating disorders. Body image is intact for people with major depression. People with schizophrenia or bipolar disorder may find this activity too threatening.

16. Answer: C

Setting a daily routine will offer a sense of control, security, and predictability. Cooking groups and crafts require multiple steps and interaction with others. The newspaper may be too stimulating and open ended.

17. Answer: D

The onset of the disease is 16 to 40 years old. A, B, and C are all true.

18. Answer: D

A Rancho Los Amigos (RLA) level of I or II means the patient appears to be sleeping or is awake but nonresponsive. PROM and sensory stimulation are appropriate treatments. A simple task is appropriate for level IV as long as it is safe, as these patients are easily agitated. Making a sandwich is a good task for level V. Community re-entry activities are best for levels VI, VII, or VIII.

19. Answer: B

Vegetative signs refer to functions related to the autonomic nervous system. Obsessive rumination is a tense state of mind related to thought content. A, C, and D are vegetative signs.

20. Answer: B

The first behavioral sign of ECT is a slight plantar extension of the feet followed by some toe, finger, or other movement.

21. Answer: A

Children from birth to 1 year old have normal pulse rates of 115 to 130. The childhood years are normal at 80 to 115. Adult years are 72 to 80 and later years are 60 to 72.

22. Answer: A

Adults can be diagnosed with mental retardation. Almost always the adult was diagnosed as a young child and carries the diagnosis into adulthood. A child or adult cannot be diagnosed with mental retardation unless born with it. Mental retardation is not a diagnosis that can be given to a child who once had normal intelligence.

23. Answer: A

A prosthesis is considered assistive or adaptive technology, not rehabilitation or educational technology. B, C, and D are all rehabilitative or educational technologies.

24. Answer: D

Arts and crafts, cooking, and shopping are problem-solving tasks. Decision making is a primary goal. A secondary effect may lead to increased self-esteem. Life management includes coping skills and self-control. These contribute to improving one's self-concept.

25. Answer: C

These are all effective OT techniques used in stress management leading to relaxation.

26. Answer: A

Thick padding often adds more pressure to the skin. Padding should only be the absolute minimum for comfort.

27. Answer: A

Confrontation is a skill used once rapport and trust have been established. It serves to point out discrepancies between thought and behavior. Empathy is the skill of fully communicating understanding of a patient's needs and feelings. Concreteness is the skill of seeking clarification, often using open-ended questions. Respect is the skill of communicating professional concern with a nonjudgmental tone.

28. Answer: A

An extended handle on the eating utensils would allow the person to feed him- or herself without moving the UE as much as traditional utensils require. A rocker knife is best used for one hand functioning. Built-up handles are best used by people with grasp problems. A spill-proof cup is best used by someone with tremors.

29. Answer: C

Children with attention deficit disorder (ADD) are more likely to be boys, have average or above average intelligence, and be impulsive. Some have hyperactivity also (ADHD). Children with ADD frequently have poor problem-solving skills.

30. Answer: B

The term "risk" suggests a negative component among the choices. Falling is the number one problem among the elderly and is related to normal changes, pathological changes, and the environment.

31. Answer: B

Undoing is the act of taking a positive action to counter an act perceived by one's ego as threatening. This is commonly seen in patients with obsessive-compulsive disorder. Projection is attributing feelings onto someone or something else, common in patients who are paranoid. Splitting is dividing people into bad or good categories, common in patients with borderline personality. Passive-aggressive is anger turned against the self.

32. Answer: B

Joint protection includes palms instead of fingers and shoulders instead of hands. Use the load carrying muscles and joints over the fine motor muscles and joints.

33. Answer: A

Pathological anxiety is an inappropriate response to a stressor in intensity or duration. B, C, and D are all normal anxiety.

34. Answer: B

A pathological fracture can indicate a tumor or osteoporosis. A greenstick fracture is seen in immature bones of children. A compound fracture is a bone broken in several places, and a comminuted fracture is a crush injury.

35. Answer: C

All flammable supplies should be kept in a ventilated, locked, metal cabinet unless the label warns differently. Hazardous materials must be used and disposed of following strict regulations. Most facilities have a hazard waste management supervisor. Check with this person concerning supplies and consider nontoxic alternatives.

36. Answer: B

Dressing the LE is the most problematic.

37. Answer: B

Rheumatoid arthritis (RA) is a classic connective tissue disease because of the inflammatory process and systemic involvement. Degenerative joint disease is noninflammatory, usually associated with osteoarthritis. RA is noted in both young and older populations and in both large and small joints.

38. Answer: C

Biomechanical frame of reference is best because of the orthopedic nature of the injury and the patient's complaint.

39. Answer: B

Good history taking may show a pattern of repetitive injury. Rapport building is important also but secondary to the nature of hand injuries. A good balance of activities and possible job changes comes later in treatment.

40. Answer: C

The MAP is a developmental assessment. The SCSIT is an evaluation of sensory integration. The MVPT is an assessment tool for visual perception with children ages 4 to 8. The Play Skills Inventory addresses observed play habits.

41. Answer: A

CHAMPUS is a health insurance plan for military personnel and their families. B, C, and D are not true.

42. Answer: A

Medicare Part B is supplementary medical insurance to Part A. It is available to persons over 65 and those with disabilities for a small monthly fee.

43. Answer: A

An incident report should be filled out immediately while details are still fresh in the therapist's mind.

44. Answer: A

As soon as the patient enters the clinic, the OTR should begin to collect data based on informal observation. Posture, facial expression, and verbalizations are an integral part of the assessment. The medical history is informative but could bias the therapist about the client.

45. Answer: B

The dysphasia patient should never "wash down" food in the mouth. Food left in the mouth should be removed with a cloth or swab. All other precautions should be followed.

46. Answer: D

Speech is adequate but content is empty or vague. Dysarthria refers to difficulty in articulation. Pressured speech refers to rapid, hard to interrupt speech. Poverty of speech refers to limited amounts of speech that may be syllabic.

47. Answer: B
Impaired thought processes should alert the OTR to the possibility of another disease.

48. Answer: A
Massage, elevation, gloves, and even dry cold packs will reduce edema, however, wet packs are contraindicated post surgery.

49. Answer: C
A narrow, shallow, and sturdy plastic spoon should be used to feed a child with reflex biting. The food will slide off easily.

50. Answer: C
Protocols differ from facility to facility. Some use 20% over resting heart rate as the stopping point of activity. Some use 120 beats per minute as the stopping rate. In either case the therapist could expect that the patient would have a pulse rate of at least 100 to 110 if engaged in strenuous exercise. Dyspnea, palpitations, and a glassy stare are all reasons to stop activity and notify the physician. The following are also signs to stop the activity and notify the physician: fatigue, faintness, dizziness, claudication pain in legs, excessive sweating, ataxic gait, irregular pulse, and high or low blood pressure.

SECTION NINE

1. Answer: A
Flexion causes pain for the person with carpal tunnel syndrome, therefore, 10° to 20° extension is the correct position.

2. Answer: A
Prism glasses are eyeglasses that bend light 90° so that a person lying on his or her back can watch television or read a book on his or her lap. B, C, and D are not true.

3. Answer: C
Scissor gait means that the hip muscles are internally rotated, in extension and adducted.

4. Answer: A
Hallucinations do not occur. Nervousness, insomnia, and headaches do occur with headaches as the most common.

5. Answer: B
Mental health treatment involves helping clients to self-disclose to family and significant others when they are ready. Helping the person deal with possible issues of rejection, guilt, shame, or anger are also roles of the occupational therapist.

6. Answer: B
Repeating the activity with more pressure allows for gradual gradation of proprioceptive input and allows the children to control the activity. Bouncing the ball over the children is both unsafe and frightening.

7. Answer: A

Binge eating is an essential feature of bulimia. B, C, and D are true.

8. Answer: D

The neck should be neutral.

9. Answer: C

Walking the tongue depressor toward the back of the tongue will desensitize the gag reflex. When possible the patient should control the tongue depressor while the therapist observes. Icing is an exercise for muscle strength. Resistance to the jaw is for jaw control. Increasing straw length is effective for sucking reflex.

10. Answer: B

If possible have the patient apply pressure himself. If not, the OT should wear a latex glove, put a gauze on the cut, and apply pressure. Return the patient to his unit and notify the nurse. Fill out the appropriate incident report forms.

11. Answer: D

Mobile arm supports are effective in proximal weakness. Although A, B, and C may be helpful, they are designed for distal weakness.

12. Answer: B

Children of teenage mothers are more likely to suffer from various problems including abuse, neglect, inadequate health, hygiene, and nutrition. A, C, and D are true.

13. Answer: D

HIV is a RNA retrovirus which is primarily present in blood, semen, and cervical and vaginal secretions. To a small degree, it is also found in tears, breast milk, and cerebrospinal fluid of infected people.

14. Answer: B

Visual concentration and ability to refocus may become enhanced in children without hearing because of dependence on visual input. Bilateral coordination, self-perception, and play skills may be problem areas.

15. Answer: A

The olfactory nerve is commonly involved in high velocity head injuries.

16. Answer: D

Timing, hot oral intake, and suppositories or digital stimulation are all important factors of bowel programs. Consistency in a daily schedule allows the bowel to adjust to a predictable routine.

17. Answer: C

The patient must move forward in the chair to have his or her center of gravity over his or her feet when he or she comes to standing.

18. Answer: C

Delays are often present due to not using hands, fear of movement, and lack of visual stimulation.

19. Answer: D

Productivity and job performance are often interrupted due to chronic pain.

20. Answer: C

The problems stated are motor functioning so the goal of increasing gross motor functioning to normal range is most appropriate. A, B, and D are possible goals for other problem areas.

21. Answer: D

MMT is a motor exam; all the others predict outcome to some degree.

22. Answer: B

Hepatitis will affect patients' ability to participate in their rehabilitation program. Diazepam (Valium) may cause seizures. Baclofen may cause hallucinations and clonidine may cause a decrease in blood pressure.

23. Answer: D

Part of energy conservation is planning ahead to pace oneself and save energy.

24. Answer: B

Using informal methods until the teenager is more comfortable with the therapist is best. Other responses are likely to further agitate the teen.

25. Answer: C

The patient with a T4 spinal cord injury can use a wheelchair with removable sides to transfer in and out of the chair. If a patient is confused or agitated, removable sides on a wheelchair would be dangerous.

26. Answer: C

The outcome of therapy, as well as the long-term cognitive ability, demands at least 2 years avoidance of alcohol. Not drinking again is preferred.

27. Answer: C

Fatigue is the biggest long-term, chronic problem. Physical and mental energy requirements are high. A, B, and D can be controlled with medication or routine procedures.

28. Answer: D

The prophylactic use of antiseizure medication can affect the patient's work in rehabilitation if there is a decrease in cognitive functioning caused by the medication.

29. Answer: B

"High-risk infant" is a term used to describe a child with body system involvement including respiratory, cardiovascular, metabolic, nutritional, immunologic, or ophthalmologic. Mental retardation is significant subaverage intellectual functioning and deficits in adaptive behavior. Failure to thrive is a disorder where children fail to grow at a normal rate for their age, gender, or race. Learning disabilities are deficits in attention, memory, reasoning, or the ability to produce responses with desired and skilled behavior.

30. Answer: D

A normal developmental behavior for teenagers is the interest in developing peer relationships.

31. Answer: D

Social structure, values, norms, and expectations all describe the cultural environment. Human environment describes individuals and groups of people. Social environment describes people with social matrix of relationships. Nonhuman environment describes conditions, things, and ideas.

32. Answer: B

Yalom is traditional psychotherapy which occupational therapists have integrated into group treatment. Fidler developed the task-oriented group. Mosey coined the developmental OT group. Ross developed the integrated five-stage group.

33. Answer: C

Increased organization is a cognitive goal.

34. Answer: A

Some psychotropic medications leave the patient sensitive to sunburn. The OTR must remind the patient to use sunscreen and protective clothing.

35. Answer: D

People with MS tend to be more mobile and therefore less likely to develop heterotropic ossification from prolonged immobility.

36. Answer: C

The hip is the most likely involved area, with the elbow second. Shoulders and fingers can be involved, but less than hips and elbows.

37. Answer: D

A patient at ACL level 1 is unable to attend to his or her basic survival needs and therefore all the activities except listening to music would be too difficult.

38. Answer: A

People with spinal cord injuries are on par with society as cardiovascular problems are the leading cause of death for all people. B, C, and D are common problems for people with spinal cord injuries but manageable with medication.

39. Answer: D

Quality assurance (QA) is a required component for all hospital or rehabilitation programs that wish to have accreditation of third party reimbursement. In addition, QA is supported by AOTA as an essential component of practice. QA is constantly being developed and requires continuous monitoring. Public schools do not require QA, however, other review systems in public schools are similar to QA in goals and methods.

40. Answer: C

Scoliosis is a lateral curvature of the spine. Kyphosis is a posterior curvature of the spine. Spina bifida is a congenital birth defect where the spinal column does not close. Rickets is a skeletal condition due to the lack of vitamin D usually seen in children.

41. Answer: A

Sacs of fluid near joint areas are called bursae. Fascia, ligaments, and tendons are also near joints but lack fluid.

42. Answer: D

While lying supine in bed, a pillow under the head and knees will reduce neck and back strain. Side-lying patients should bend their knees and use a pillow to support the head. Watch for hip and neck contractures if the patient is bedridden for long periods.

43. Answer: C

A demonstration may help the patient understand what it is that you want him to do. A, B, and D will only further agitate the patient.

44. Answer: A

Patients dealing with or recovering from cancer have diverse needs, often including most of the components and areas of Uniform Terminology. Prognosis, treatments, and medications are the expertise of the physician. Encourage the patient to ask her doctor. If she is unable to do this independently, assist her in developing the needed skills or refer her to someone who can advocate for her.

45. Answer: B

This is a monitoring plan. A, C, and D are all indicators of quality programs.

46. Answer: B

Critical periods for brain development extend from pregnancy to early childhood when rapid growth and development occurs.

47. Answer: B

Sexual counseling is a component of occupational therapy. Competency and success is based on the OTR's personal awareness, basic knowledge, and interpersonal skills. The OTR needs to feel comfortable communicating with patients about their sexual issues and therefore must be comfortable with his or her own sexuality.

48. Answer: B

Different sexual positions are helpful in relieving stress on joints. A, C, and D would be ineffective in addressing the issue.

49. Answer: C

While some evidence suggests that stereotyped behaviors may be lessened or interrupted, there is no evidence to show sensory stimulation can eliminate the underlying cause of behavior.

50. Answer: B

Hand preference is usually established by school age.

SECTION IV
Life After the Exam

Chapter Seven
Life After the Exam

Karen Sladyk and Julie Seethaler

WAITING FOR THE RESULTS

Many occupational therapy students have said to us that waiting for the exam results is almost as hard as studying for the exam itself. Generally you can expect the results in approximately 4 weeks. Do not listen to rumors of how the results will look when you get them. We have heard that if the envelope has your name with OTR next to it, you passed. We have also heard that if the envelope is thick, you passed. These rumors are not true. The only way to know if you passed the exam is to open the envelope.

WHAT IF YOU DID NOT PASS?

Although the number of people who do not pass the exam to become occupational therapists is small, the reality is that some students will not pass and it may be you. There are many reasons why students do not pass the exam. When they took the exam, some had major stressors in their life, such as a family illness or recent death. There are students who did well in school but may not be good test takers. Some students did not prepare for the exam by reviewing their weaker areas but simply reviewed their comfortable areas. Finally, there are those students who did not pass the exam for any clear-cut reason. Whatever the reason, it is our experience that you should not spend a lot of time ruminating over the fact that you did not pass. Of course, we realize that this is easy for us to say and the bottom line is that not passing the exam hurts a lot.

WHAT TO DO FIRST

If you have accepted a job offer or have already begun working, you will have to notify your employer. If possible, speak to the director of occupational therapy. The director will understand your problem better than the personnel department. Depending on the licensure laws in your state, you may be able to keep your job working as an occupational therapy aide or rehabilitation associate while studying for the next exam. Keep in mind that you do not want to practice occupational therapy until you have passed the exam due to liability concerns.

Other than the licensing board in your state who will receive your scores from the NBCOT, no one else has access to your exam. We recommend that you share information about not passing with those who can be supportive as you study for the next exam. It is important to know that your school does not know who did not pass the exam unless you tell them.

After you have notified your employer, you should check with the appropriate people for further information about working and studying. These people may include:

- The testing center for hand correcting the exam you took.
- The program director at your school.
- The state licensing board for occupational therapists for further questions.
- Your friends from school.
- Other OTRs who can help you study weak areas.
- Other professors you found helpful or supportive in school.

The company who administers the exam offers an option to hand correct your exam for a small fee. Although the chances that the machine did not correctly score the exam are extremely rare, you may feel better knowing that you have investigated every route available to you.

Lastly, we would like to discuss the emotional aspects of not passing the exam. It is our experience that this is a strong factor on how students cope with studying for the next exam. Not passing the exam the first time around will seem like a major loss in your life. It is expected that you deal with this loss in the same way that people usually deal with stressors. You can expect feelings of shock, anger, depression, and bargaining at first. Acceptance and coping will come later. Again, it is our experience that everyone does cope and is able to sit for the next exam. Since the exam is given every 6 months, you will have about 5 months to prepare for the next exam. Generally, this is enough time to develop coping skills. If coping is more difficult for you, seek professional help to deal with stress. We believe that counseling or therapy is one of the best treats you can give yourself. Do not be afraid or feel guilty for seeking professional help. Your college counseling center can provide you with a list of local supports.

HOW TO GET GOING AGAIN

Keep in mind that you are not the only one who has not passed the exam this time. You are not the first one, nor will you be the last one. It is important to keep things in perspective to increase your ability to cope. The following is a letter from an OTR who did not pass the exam the first time.

To all students and future occupational therapists:

At this point in my life, I think it is important for me to share my personal story with you. My teachers in college would have described me as an above average student, but I worked hard to be there. During my last affiliation, with much resistance and procrastination, I began to study for the OT boards. When the day arrived to take the exam, I was quite anxious. When I walked out, it was hard to know how I did but I was confident I had passed. Ironically, I consoled a friend and classmate who was confident she had failed.

After waiting 4 long weeks, I received the results. I had failed. I kept staring at the words "you did not meet the requirements..." Not only that but there was an address to reapply.

I was supposed to be celebrating. They told us in school that "everyone passes" (or at least that was my perception). Despite many sad days and feeling unmotivated to try again, I got the books out and studied. When I looked back, I realized that I had studied the information I knew and was comfortable with instead of focusing on my weak areas of practice.

This time I did my preparation differently. I studied in a group. I reviewed with peers. I used an outdated review book that provided me with structure. Lastly, I studied for many hours on my own. I focused only on my areas of weakness.

One thing that is important to mention is that I always had a tremendous amount of support from my family and friends. With all the support, studying, and courage to try again, I finally passed the exam the following year.

Although statistics show a low percentage rate for failing the exam, it does happen. It happened to me. My best advice is don't give up. Do your best and use supportive people to help you through the challenge. Although initially it was devastating, in the end it was a tremendous personal growth experience for me. I am currently practicing occupational therapy in an area that I enjoy and I'm proud to be an OTR.

My goal with this letter is to let everyone know that if you fail, you are not a failure. Do not give up even though you will have a strong desire to do so.

Best wishes to everyone,

J.T.

MAKING A NEW PLAN

Once you are ready to start studying again, it is important to develop a personalized plan of action. Chapter Two of this book took you through the planning process. As an OT who did not pass the exam the first time, you may need some additional plans in place. Look carefully at what caused difficulty the first time; however, understand that you may never know for sure what went wrong on the first exam. Globally review all your class notes and focus on weak areas of practice.

Understand that periods of anxiety and sadness may creep back on you as you prepare to take the exam again. If you are a person who experiences test anxiety, taking the exam a second time will likely cause much stress. Consider a relaxation exercise or visualize yourself calmly taking the exam and passing. Begin and end each study period with a visualization of you taking the exam and all the information you have studied flowing from your brain, down your arm, and onto the answer sheet. Feel yourself calm, relaxed, and happy.

IF YOU DO NOT PASS AGAIN

Should you not pass the exam for a second time, you need to know what options are available to you. We know some great practicing occupational therapists who have experienced this challenge. Again, do not give up. If in your heart you know that occupational therapy is for you, do a thorough self-assessment of what went wrong, seek the help you need, and prepare to take the exam again.

SUMMARY

Finding out that you did not pass the OTR exam will bring many emotional and cognitive challenges to you. Developing coping skills and preparing for the exam often will lead to passing the exam the next time. A thorough self-assessment of what went wrong the first time will help you develop an action plan. Notifying your employer if you are working and developing a support network of people who can help you study may be an effective way of coping with the challenges. Learning and using relaxation exercises may also be helpful. Whatever your options, do not give up—develop your resources and use your supports.

Appendices

Appendix A
Annotated Bibliography

Allen, C. K., Earhart, C. A., & Blue, T. (1992). *Occupational therapy treatment goals for the physically and cognitively disabled.* Bethesda, MD: American Occupational Therapy Association.
Provides information on cognitive function, evaluation, and instruments. Performance analysis is reviewed in detail and suggestions for treatment are provided.

Asher, I. E. (1989). *An annotated index of occupational therapy evaluation tools.* Bethesda, MD: American Occupational Therapy Association.
Provides an annotated list of more than 100 assessments commonly used in occupational therapy. Each assessment summary includes target population, statistical information, and assessment sources.

Bonder, B. R. (1995). *Psychopathology and function* (2nd ed.). Thorofare, NJ: SLACK Inc.
Major psychiatric disorders are described according to symptomatology, etiology, and prognosis with implications for function and treatment. A description of occupational therapy treatment with reference to Uniform Terminology is provided within each classification.

Borg, B., & Bruce, M. A. (1991). *The group system.* Thorofare, NJ: SLACK Inc.
Provides discussion of the small therapeutic group, its relationship to occupational therapy, and comparison to system theories and group dynamic theories. A major goal of the presenters is to give practical information to group leaders through examples.

Bruce, M. A., & Borg, B. (1993). *Frames of reference in psychosocial occupational therapy* (2nd ed.). Thorofare, NJ: SLACK Inc.
Six frames of reference in psychiatric occupational therapy are discussed in detail including developmental, cognitive, cognitive behavioral, object relations, behavioral, and occupational behavioral. Additional information on organic mental disorders and the suicidal patient is included.

Christiansen, C., & Baum, C. (1997). *Occupational therapy: Enabling function and well-being* (2nd ed.). Thorofare, NJ: SLACK Inc.
Provides framework of occupational therapy and identifies the links between theory and practice. Discusses reasoning and decision-making processes necessary for competent occupational therapy practice.

Cole, M. (1993). *Group dynamics in occupational therapy.* Thorofare, NJ: SLACK Inc.
Provides an explanation of the theoretical base of occupational therapy group treatment. Organized as a workbook, this book provides guidelines and suggestions for occupational therapists and students to use and implement group process in treatment.

Dunn, W. (1991). *Pediatric occupational therapy.* Thorofare, NJ: SLACK Inc.

Discusses both service and support models of pediatric occupational therapy referral, screening, assessment, and treatment. Includes family, educators, and medical perspectives. Assessments commonly used are discussed, as well as documentation and marketing.

Fiorentino, M. R. (1972). *Normal and abnormal development.* Springfield, IL: Charles C. Thomas Publishing.

A classic resource on the influence of primitive reflexes on motor development, this text provides an orientation to the developmental motor milestones in the normal child. In addition, examples of abnormal development seen in cerebral palsy are also featured.

Frender, G. (1990). *Learning to learn.* Nashville, TN: Incentives Publications.

A hands-on guide of practical hints, methods, tips, procedures, and tools for learning how to learn. Includes topics such as learning styles, organizational skills, memory, time management, and test-taking skills.

Gilfoyle, E. M., Grady, A. P., & Moore, J. C. (1990). *Children adapt.* Thorofare, NJ: SLACK Inc.

The theory of sensorimotor-sensory development is presented with nervous system and spatiotemporal adaptation highlighted. Developmental sequences are used in treatment to gain skilled performance.

Greene, L. J., & Jones-Bamman, L. (1985). *Getting smart: The study skills improvement program.* Belmont, CA: Fearon Janus.

A study skills system designed to teach how to function more efficiently in school. Step-by-step activities include worksheets on evaluating current study habits, becoming organized, improving comprehension, and how to take tests with better results.

Hansen, R., & Atchison, B. (1993). *Conditions in occupational therapy: Effects on occupational performance.* Baltimore, MD: Williams & Wilkins.

Pathophysiology of major conditions most frequently seen in occupational therapy clinics are reviewed. Diagnostic test, medical management, and occupational performance perspectives are addressed in case study reviews.

Hemphill, B. (1988). *Mental health assessment in occupational therapy.* Thorofare, NJ: SLACK Inc.

Provides in-depth discussion on several commonly used assessments in psychiatric occupational therapy, including assessments for independent living skills and work. In addition, a detailed chapter on the interview process is included.

Hopkins, H., & Smith, H. (1993). *Willard and Spackman's occupational therapy* (8th ed.). Philadelphia, PA: J. B. Lippincott.

A resource for general professional issues including occupational therapy history, philosophy, occupational science, 11 frames of reference, Uniform Terminology, and practice issues across the lifespan.

Jacobs, K. (1997). *Quick reference dictionary for occupational therapy.* Thorofare, NJ: SLACK Inc.
Provides definitions of occupational therapy terms, concepts, and conditions, as well as informative appendices.

Joe, B. E., ed. (1991). *Quality assurance in occupational therapy.* Bethesda, MD: American Occupational Therapy Association.
Three models for practitioners to develop quality assurance plans are provided. Historical overview of quality assurance, as well as numerous examples of plans, are also included.

Kaplan, H. I., Sadock, B. J., & Grebb, J. A. (1994). *Synopsis of psychiatry.* Baltimore, MD: Williams & Wilkins.
Provides an extensive reference and explanation of the DSM-IV including all psychiatric classifications from various theoretical models. Clinical explanations and classic treatment are described in detail.

Kaplan, K. L. (1988). *Directive group therapy.* Thorofare, NJ: SLACK Inc.
Provides concepts and practical guidance to use of this therapy model designed specifically for the person functioning at a minimal level.

Kiernat, J. M. (1991). *Occupational therapy and the older adult: A clinical manual.* Gaithersburg, MD: Aspen Publications.
This text reviews aging, functional changes, and adaptation of adults over 65 years. Treatment information includes the role of fitness, empowerment, preventing falls, and cognition aspects. Medicare is fully reviewed. Both community and long-term treatment are discussed in detail including assessment, treatment, and discharge planning.

Lang, S. M., ed. (1994). *AOTCB study guide for the OTR certification examination.* Bethesda, MD: American Occupational Therapy Certification Board.
Explains the certification process and provides suggestions for taking the OTR exam. Includes 50 sample questions and answer explanations.

Leonard, P. C. (1990). *Quick and easy medical terminology.* Philadelphia, PA: W. B. Saunders Co.
A self-study test that provides a repetition and quiz format for learning medical terminology.

Lewis, S. C. (1989). *Elder care in occupational therapy.* Thorofare, NJ: SLACK Inc.
A detailed text on normal development and challenges of aging. Disease process and treatment are discussed including discussion on death and dying. Medicare laws, rules, and funding are fully described.

Millen, H. M. (1978). *Body mechanics and safe transfer techniques.* Detroit, MI: Aronsson Printing.
A practical guide with numerous photographs of proper body mechanics and transfers of patients. Discusses special techniques for heavy transfers and emergency transfers.

Norkin, C., & Levangie, P. (1992). *Joint structure and function: A comprehensive analysis.* Philadelphia, PA: F. A. Davis Co.
Presents basic theory of joint structure and muscle action necessary to understanding both normal and abnormal function. A review of biomechanics is included.

Pedretti, L. (1990). *Occupational therapy skills for physical dysfunction.* St. Louis, MO: Mosby.
A basic level reference for clinicians, this text provides the application techniques for the treatment of adults with acquired physical dysfunction. Occupational therapy evaluation and treatment issues are addressed.

Reed, K. L. (1991). *Quick reference to occupational therapy.* Gaithersburg, MD: Aspen Publications.
An extensive review of common disorders across the age span and disability practice. Information on the cause, assessment, and treatment is provided in outline format. Precautions and outcomes are described. References and further readings specific to the disorders are provided.

Simmons, P. L., & Mullins, L. (1981). *Acute psychiatric care.* Thorofare, NJ: SLACK Inc.
A practical guide to group exercises in daily living skills. Includes suggestions in leisure, assertiveness, employment, money management, and discharge planning.

Sladyk, K. (1997). *OT student primer: A guide to college success.* Thorofare, NJ: SLACK Inc.
Basic OT concepts and techniques reviewed.

Sonbuchner, G. M. (1991). *Finding your best learning styles and study environment.* Rochelle Park, NJ: Peoples Publishing Group.
A booklet designed to determine one's best learning style. Strategies are presented to enhance particular learning strengths.

Sonbuchner, G. M. (1991). *Time management.* Rochelle Park, NJ: Peoples Publishing Group.
A booklet presenting basic time management strategies including time-saving tips, making better use of study time, and keeping track of things that need to be done.

Trombly, C. (1989). *Occupational therapy for physical dysfunction.* Baltimore, MD: Williams & Wilkins.
Principles of practice in adult physical dysfunction are featured. Major diagnostic areas are covered with focus on assessment and treatment. Numerous photographs illustrate basic techniques.

Yalom, I. D. (1985). *The theory and practice of group psychotherapy.* New York, NY: Basic Books.
Provides a scholarly review of various group therapy models based on recent developments in the field, as well as the author's expertise with clinical syndromes.

Zoltan, B. (1996). *Vision, perception, and cognition: A manual for the evaluation and treatment of the neurologically impaired adult* (3rd ed.). Thorofare, NJ: SLACK Inc.
Manual defines and outlines the theoretical basis of visual, perceptual, and cognitive deficits. Evaluation procedures and treatment are also identified.

Philadelphia

Appendix B
Helpful Abbreviations

The following is a list of abbreviations you may find helpful. You do not need to commit them to memory for the OTR exam, however, a working knowledge of them is useful.

ADA	Americans with Disabilities Act
ADL	activities of daily living
AIDS	acquired immune deficiency syndrome
AOTA	American Occupational Therapy Association
AOTF	American Occupational Therapy Foundation
AROM	active range of motion
CARF	Commission of Accredited Rehabilitation Facilities
COPD	chronic obstructive pulmonary disease
COTA	certified occupational therapy assistant
COTE	Comprehensive Occupational Therapy Evaluation
CVA	cerebral vascular accident
DIP	distal interphalangeal
DRG	diagnosis related groups
ECT	electroconvulsive therapy
FOR	frame of reference
HMO	health maintenance organization
JCAHO	Joint Commission on Accreditation of Healthcare Organizations
MCP	metacarpal phalangeal
MMT	manual muscle test
MORE	measurable, observable, realistic, explicit
NBCOT	National Board for Certification in Occupational Therapy
OBRA	Omnibus Budget Reconciliation Act
OT	occupational therapy, occupational therapist
OTR	occupational therapist, registered

PIP	proximal interphalangeal
POMR	problem-oriented medical record
PROM	passive range of motion
ROM	range of motion
SOAP	subjective, objective, assessment, plan
SSI/SSD	Social Security Insurance/Social Security Disability

Appendix C
Selected Study Guide References

The following books are suggested for learning more about how to study. This list is selected references only. Endorsement is not to be construed and the authors recommend that the student base his or her selection of books on personal strengths and weaknesses.

Apps, J. W. (1982). *Study skills for adults returning to school.* New York: McGraw Hill.

Armstrong, W. H. (1983). *Study tactics.* Woodbury, NY: Barron's Educational Inc.

Coman, M. J. (1990). *How to improve your study skills.* Lincolnwood, IL: VGM Career.

Davies, D. (1986). *Maximizing examination performance.* New York: Nichols Publishing.

Feder, B. (1979). *The complete guide to taking tests.* Englewood Cliffs, NJ: Prentice Hall.

Frender, G. (1990). *Learning to learn.* Nashville, TN: Incentives Publications.

Semones, J. (1991). *Effective study skills.* Fort Worth, TX: Semones Publishing.

Appendix D
Answer Sheets

EXAMINATION(S) YOU ARE TAKING	
CITY	STATE

1 A① B② C③ D④   21 A① B② C③ D④   41 A① B② C③ D④
2 A① B② C③ D④   22 A① B② C③ D④   42 A① B② C③ D④
3 A① B② C③ D④   23 A① B② C③ D④   43 A① B② C③ D④
4 A① B② C③ D④   24 A① B② C③ D④   44 A① B② C③ D④
5 A① B② C③ D④   25 A① B② C③ D④   45 A① B② C③ D④
6 A① B② C③ D④   26 A① B② C③ D④   46 A① B② C③ D④
7 A① B② C③ D④   27 A① B② C③ D④   47 A① B② C③ D④
8 A① B② C③ D④   28 A① B② C③ D④   48 A① B② C③ D④
9 A① B② C③ D④   29 A① B② C③ D④   49 A① B② C③ D④
10 A① B② C③ D④   30 A① B② C③ D④   50 A① B② C③ D④
11 A① B② C③ D④   31 A① B② C③ D④
12 A① B② C③ D④   32 A① B② C③ D④
13 A① B② C③ D④   33 A① B② C③ D④
14 A① B② C③ D④   34 A① B② C③ D④
15 A① B② C③ D④   35 A① B② C③ D④
16 A① B② C③ D④   36 A① B② C③ D④
17 A① B② C③ D④   37 A① B② C③ D④
18 A① B② C③ D④   38 A① B② C③ D④
19 A① B② C③ D④   39 A① B② C③ D④
20 A① B② C③ D④   40 A① B② C③ D④

EXAMINATION(S) YOU ARE TAKING	
CITY	STATE

1 A B C D ① ② ③ ④	21 A B C D ① ② ③ ④	41 A B C D ① ② ③ ④
2 A B C D ① ② ③ ④	22 A B C D ① ② ③ ④	42 A B C D ① ② ③ ④
3 A B C D ① ② ③ ④	23 A B C D ① ② ③ ④	43 A B C D ① ② ③ ④
4 A B C D ① ② ③ ④	24 A B C D ① ② ③ ④	44 A B C D ① ② ③ ④
5 A B C D ① ② ③ ④	25 A B C D ① ② ③ ④	45 A B C D ① ② ③ ④
6 A B C D ① ② ③ ④	26 A B C D ① ② ③ ④	46 A B C D ① ② ③ ④
7 A B C D ① ② ③ ④	27 A B C D ① ② ③ ④	47 A B C D ① ② ③ ④
8 A B C D ① ② ③ ④	28 A B C D ① ② ③ ④	48 A B C D ① ② ③ ④
9 A B C D ① ② ③ ④	29 A B C D ① ② ③ ④	49 A B C D ① ② ③ ④
10 A B C D ① ② ③ ④	30 A B C D ① ② ③ ④	50 A B C D ① ② ③ ④
11 A B C D ① ② ③ ④	31 A B C D ① ② ③ ④	
12 A B C D ① ② ③ ④	32 A B C D ① ② ③ ④	
13 A B C D ① ② ③ ④	33 A B C D ① ② ③ ④	
14 A B C D ① ② ③ ④	34 A B C D ① ② ③ ④	
15 A B C D ① ② ③ ④	35 A B C D ① ② ③ ④	
16 A B C D ① ② ③ ④	36 A B C D ① ② ③ ④	
17 A B C D ① ② ③ ④	37 A B C D ① ② ③ ④	
18 A B C D ① ② ③ ④	38 A B C D ① ② ③ ④	
19 A B C D ① ② ③ ④	39 A B C D ① ② ③ ④	
20 A B C D ① ② ③ ④	40 A B C D ① ② ③ ④	

EXAMINATION(S) YOU ARE TAKING	
CITY	STATE

1 A① B② C③ D④   21 A① B② C③ D④   41 A① B② C③ D④

2 A① B② C③ D④   22 A① B② C③ D④   42 A① B② C③ D④

3 A① B② C③ D④   23 A① B② C③ D④   43 A① B② C③ D④

4 A① B② C③ D④   24 A① B② C③ D④   44 A① B② C③ D④

5 A① B② C③ D④   25 A① B② C③ D④   45 A① B② C③ D④

6 A① B② C③ D④   26 A① B② C③ D④   46 A① B② C③ D④

7 A① B② C③ D④   27 A① B② C③ D④   47 A① B② C③ D④

8 A① B② C③ D④   28 A① B② C③ D④   48 A① B② C③ D④

9 A① B② C③ D④   29 A① B② C③ D④   49 A① B② C③ D④

10 A① B② C③ D④   30 A① B② C③ D④   50 A① B② C③ D④

11 A① B② C③ D④   31 A① B② C③ D④

12 A① B② C③ D④   32 A① B② C③ D④

13 A① B② C③ D④   33 A① B② C③ D④

14 A① B② C③ D④   34 A① B② C③ D④

15 A① B② C③ D④   35 A① B② C③ D④

16 A① B② C③ D④   36 A① B② C③ D④

17 A① B② C③ D④   37 A① B② C③ D④

18 A① B② C③ D④   38 A① B② C③ D④

19 A① B② C③ D④   39 A① B② C③ D④

20 A① B② C③ D④   40 A① B② C③ D④

EXAMINATION(S) YOU ARE TAKING	
CITY	STATE

1 A① B② C③ D④   21 A① B② C③ D④   41 A① B② C③ D④

2 A① B② C③ D④   22 A① B② C③ D④   42 A① B② C③ D④

3 A① B② C③ D④   23 A① B② C③ D④   43 A① B② C③ D④

4 A① B② C③ D④   24 A① B② C③ D④   44 A① B② C③ D④

5 A① B② C③ D④   25 A① B② C③ D④   45 A① B② C③ D④

6 A① B② C③ D④   26 A① B② C③ D④   46 A① B② C③ D④

7 A① B② C③ D④   27 A① B② C③ D④   47 A① B② C③ D④

8 A① B② C③ D④   28 A① B② C③ D④   48 A① B② C③ D④

9 A① B② C③ D④   29 A① B② C③ D④   49 A① B② C③ D④

10 A① B② C③ D④   30 A① B② C③ D④   50 A① B② C③ D④

11 A① B② C③ D④   31 A① B② C③ D④

12 A① B② C③ D④   32 A① B② C③ D④

13 A① B② C③ D④   33 A① B② C③ D④

14 A① B② C③ D④   34 A① B② C③ D④

15 A① B② C③ D④   35 A① B② C③ D④

16 A① B② C③ D④   36 A① B② C③ D④

17 A① B② C③ D④   37 A① B② C③ D④

18 A① B② C③ D④   38 A① B② C③ D④

19 A① B② C③ D④   39 A① B② C③ D④

20 A① B② C③ D④   40 A① B② C③ D④

EXAMINATION(S) YOU ARE TAKING	
CITY	STATE

	A	B	C	D			A	B	C	D			A	B	C	D
1	A ①	B ②	C ③	D ④		21	A ①	B ②	C ③	D ④		41	A ①	B ②	C ③	D ④
2	A ①	B ②	C ③	D ④		22	A ①	B ②	C ③	D ④		42	A ①	B ②	C ③	D ④
3	A ①	B ②	C ③	D ④		23	A ①	B ②	C ③	D ④		43	A ①	B ②	C ③	D ④
4	A ①	B ②	C ③	D ④		24	A ①	B ②	C ③	D ④		44	A ①	B ②	C ③	D ④
5	A ①	B ②	C ③	D ④		25	A ①	B ②	C ③	D ④		45	A ①	B ②	C ③	D ④
6	A ①	B ②	C ③	D ④		26	A ①	B ②	C ③	D ④		46	A ①	B ②	C ③	D ④
7	A ①	B ②	C ③	D ④		27	A ①	B ②	C ③	D ④		47	A ①	B ②	C ③	D ④
8	A ①	B ②	C ③	D ④		28	A ①	B ②	C ③	D ④		48	A ①	B ②	C ③	D ④
9	A ①	B ②	C ③	D ④		29	A ①	B ②	C ③	D ④		49	A ①	B ②	C ③	D ④
10	A ①	B ②	C ③	D ④		30	A ①	B ②	C ③	D ④		50	A ①	B ②	C ③	D ④
11	A ①	B ②	C ③	D ④		31	A ①	B ②	C ③	D ④						
12	A ①	B ②	C ③	D ④		32	A ①	B ②	C ③	D ④						
13	A ①	B ②	C ③	D ④		33	A ①	B ②	C ③	D ④						
14	A ①	B ②	C ③	D ④		34	A ①	B ②	C ③	D ④						
15	A ①	B ②	C ③	D ④		35	A ①	B ②	C ③	D ④						
16	A ①	B ②	C ③	D ④		36	A ①	B ②	C ③	D ④						
17	A ①	B ②	C ③	D ④		37	A ①	B ②	C ③	D ④						
18	A ①	B ②	C ③	D ④		38	A ①	B ②	C ③	D ④						
19	A ①	B ②	C ③	D ④		39	A ①	B ②	C ③	D ④						
20	A ①	B ②	C ③	D ④		40	A ①	B ②	C ③	D ④						

EXAMINATION(S) YOU ARE TAKING	
CITY	STATE

1	A ① B ② C ③ D ④	21	A ① B ② C ③ D ④	41 A ① B ② C ③ D ④
2	A ① B ② C ③ D ④	22	A ① B ② C ③ D ④	42 A ① B ② C ③ D ④
3	A ① B ② C ③ D ④	23	A ① B ② C ③ D ④	43 A ① B ② C ③ D ④
4	A ① B ② C ③ D ④	24	A ① B ② C ③ D ④	44 A ① B ② C ③ D ④
5	A ① B ② C ③ D ④	25	A ① B ② C ③ D ④	45 A ① B ② C ③ D ④
6	A ① B ② C ③ D ④	26	A ① B ② C ③ D ④	46 A ① B ② C ③ D ④
7	A ① B ② C ③ D ④	27	A ① B ② C ③ D ④	47 A ① B ② C ③ D ④
8	A ① B ② C ③ D ④	28	A ① B ② C ③ D ④	48 A ① B ② C ③ D ④
9	A ① B ② C ③ D ④	29	A ① B ② C ③ D ④	49 A ① B ② C ③ D ④
10	A ① B ② C ③ D ④	30	A ① B ② C ③ D ④	50 A ① B ② C ③ D ④
11	A ① B ② C ③ D ④	31	A ① B ② C ③ D ④	
12	A ① B ② C ③ D ④	32	A ① B ② C ③ D ④	
13	A ① B ② C ③ D ④	33	A ① B ② C ③ D ④	
14	A ① B ② C ③ D ④	34	A ① B ② C ③ D ④	
15	A ① B ② C ③ D ④	35	A ① B ② C ③ D ④	
16	A ① B ② C ③ D ④	36	A ① B ② C ③ D ④	
17	A ① B ② C ③ D ④	37	A ① B ② C ③ D ④	
18	A ① B ② C ③ D ④	38	A ① B ② C ③ D ④	
19	A ① B ② C ③ D ④	39	A ① B ② C ③ D ④	
20	A ① B ② C ③ D ④	40	A ① B ② C ③ D ④	

EXAMINATION(S) YOU ARE TAKING	
CITY	STATE

1	A ① B ② C ③ D ④	21	A ① B ② C ③ D ④	41	A ① B ② C ③ D ④
2	A ① B ② C ③ D ④	22	A ① B ② C ③ D ④	42	A ① B ② C ③ D ④
3	A ① B ② C ③ D ④	23	A ① B ② C ③ D ④	43	A ① B ② C ③ D ④
4	A ① B ② C ③ D ④	24	A ① B ② C ③ D ④	44	A ① B ② C ③ D ④
5	A ① B ② C ③ D ④	25	A ① B ② C ③ D ④	45	A ① B ② C ③ D ④
6	A ① B ② C ③ D ④	26	A ① B ② C ③ D ④	46	A ① B ② C ③ D ④
7	A ① B ② C ③ D ④	27	A ① B ② C ③ D ④	47	A ① B ② C ③ D ④
8	A ① B ② C ③ D ④	28	A ① B ② C ③ D ④	48	A ① B ② C ③ D ④
9	A ① B ② C ③ D ④	29	A ① B ② C ③ D ④	49	A ① B ② C ③ D ④
10	A ① B ② C ③ D ④	30	A ① B ② C ③ D ④	50	A ① B ② C ③ D ④
11	A ① B ② C ③ D ④	31	A ① B ② C ③ D ④		
12	A ① B ② C ③ D ④	32	A ① B ② C ③ D ④		
13	A ① B ② C ③ D ④	33	A ① B ② C ③ D ④		
14	A ① B ② C ③ D ④	34	A ① B ② C ③ D ④		
15	A ① B ② C ③ D ④	35	A ① B ② C ③ D ④		
16	A ① B ② C ③ D ④	36	A ① B ② C ③ D ④		
17	A ① B ② C ③ D ④	37	A ① B ② C ③ D ④		
18	A ① B ② C ③ D ④	38	A ① B ② C ③ D ④		
19	A ① B ② C ③ D ④	39	A ① B ② C ③ D ④		
20	A ① B ② C ③ D ④	40	A ① B ② C ③ D ④		

EXAMINATION(S) YOU ARE TAKING	
CITY	STATE

1 A① B② C③ D④ 21 A① B② C③ D④ 41 A① B② C③ D④

2 A① B② C③ D④ 22 A① B② C③ D④ 42 A① B② C③ D④

3 A① B② C③ D④ 23 A① B② C③ D④ 43 A① B② C③ D④

4 A① B② C③ D④ 24 A① B② C③ D④ 44 A① B② C③ D④

5 A① B② C③ D④ 25 A① B② C③ D④ 45 A① B② C③ D④

6 A① B② C③ D④ 26 A① B② C③ D④ 46 A① B② C③ D④

7 A① B② C③ D④ 27 A① B② C③ D④ 47 A① B② C③ D④

8 A① B② C③ D④ 28 A① B② C③ D④ 48 A① B② C③ D④

9 A① B② C③ D④ 29 A① B② C③ D④ 49 A① B② C③ D④

10 A① B② C③ D④ 30 A① B② C③ D④ 50 A① B② C③ D④

11 A① B② C③ D④ 31 A① B② C③ D④

12 A① B② C③ D④ 32 A① B② C③ D④

13 A① B② C③ D④ 33 A① B② C③ D④

14 A① B② C③ D④ 34 A① B② C③ D④

15 A① B② C③ D④ 35 A① B② C③ D④

16 A① B② C③ D④ 36 A① B② C③ D④

17 A① B② C③ D④ 37 A① B② C③ D④

18 A① B② C③ D④ 38 A① B② C③ D④

19 A① B② C③ D④ 39 A① B② C③ D④

20 A① B② C③ D④ 40 A① B② C③ D④

EXAMINATION(S) YOU ARE TAKING	
CITY	STATE

1 A① B② C③ D④ 21 A① B② C③ D④ 41 A① B② C③ D④

2 A① B② C③ D④ 22 A① B② C③ D④ 42 A① B② C③ D④

3 A① B② C③ D④ 23 A① B② C③ D④ 43 A① B② C③ D④

4 A① B② C③ D④ 24 A① B② C③ D④ 44 A① B② C③ D④

5 A① B② C③ D④ 25 A① B② C③ D④ 45 A① B② C③ D④

6 A① B② C③ D④ 26 A① B② C③ D④ 46 A① B② C③ D④

7 A① B② C③ D④ 27 A① B② C③ D④ 47 A① B② C③ D④

8 A① B② C③ D④ 28 A① B② C③ D④ 48 A① B② C③ D④

9 A① B② C③ D④ 29 A① B② C③ D④ 49 A① B② C③ D④

10 A① B② C③ D④ 30 A① B② C③ D④ 50 A① B② C③ D④

11 A① B② C③ D④ 31 A① B② C③ D④

12 A① B② C③ D④ 32 A① B② C③ D④

13 A① B② C③ D④ 33 A① B② C③ D④

14 A① B② C③ D④ 34 A① B② C③ D④

15 A① B② C③ D④ 35 A① B② C③ D④

16 A① B② C③ D④ 36 A① B② C③ D④

17 A① B② C③ D④ 37 A① B② C③ D④

18 A① B② C③ D④ 38 A① B② C③ D④

19 A① B② C③ D④ 39 A① B② C③ D④

20 A① B② C③ D④ 40 A① B② C③ D④

Appendix E
Authors' Feedback Form

The authors need your help!

As the consumer of this study guide, you have valuable information you can provide the authors of this book. Please take a few minutes after you are finished studying with this book and tell us what was good and what needs improvement. Future occupational therapy students will greatly benefit from your insight.

1. Please list the sections of the book you found helpful.

2. What was the most helpful?

3. Could you briefly tell us why it was the most helpful?

4. Please list the sections of the book you feel need improvement.

5. What was the least helpful?

6. Could you briefly tell us why it was the least helpful?

7. Where or how did you find this book?

8. Do you think this book should be an optional textbook in OTR school?

9. Do you think this book should be a required textbook in OTR school?

Is there anything else you would like to tell us?

About you:

Your age:

Your gender:

Circle the type of degree you have or will earn:
BA   BS   Post BS Certificate   MA   MS   MOT

Mail the completed form to Karen Sladyk, PhD, OTR/L, in care of SLACK Incorporated, 6900 Grove Road, Thorofare, NJ 08086-9447.

Index